Making the Words
Stand Still

DONALD E. LYMAN

Making the Words Stand Still

A Master Teacher
Tells How to Overcome
Specific Learning Disability,
Dyslexia, and
Old-Fashioned Word Blindness

Foreword by Robert S. Sloat

Houghton Mifflin Company • Boston • 1986

Library of Congress Cataloging in Publication Data

Lyman, Donald E.
 Making the words stand still.

 Includes index.
 1. Learning disabilities. 2. Learning disabled
children. 3. Lyman, Donald E. 4. Teachers of
handicapped children — United States — Biography.
5. Dyslexic children — United States — Biography.
I. Title.
LC4704.L96 1986   371.9   85-14550
ISBN 0-395-36219-9

Printed in the United States of America

S 10 9 8 7 6 5 4 3 2 1

Book design by Victoria Hartman

To all with special learning abilities,
especially my daughter,
Jennifer

The asking of a question with passionate concern for its answer, a concern which demands life investment, suggests a door which will sooner or later be found. Whether it is successfully opened to the public is another matter, but if a current world view can accommodate a new synthesis, the new idea may prove to be the case.

— *Joseph Chilton Pearce*

Contents

KAREN'S WORDS . . .

"WORDS HAVE ALWAYS BULLIED ME around. I have been afraid of words as long as I can remember. Not afraid of saying them, but seeing them and hearing them. Maybe I've been afraid of thinking them too because they never seemed comfortable inside my head as pictures, music and feelings did.

"I was mad when they decided to call me learning disabled. Maybe I was word disabled, but learning was no problem for me.

"Lately words haven't been scaring me as much. In fact, they hardly scare me at all. I've been practicing with them a whole lot more than I ever did and I'm getting better with them, but that's not the reason I can stand up to them now. I can do this because I've grown smart enough to understand that disability is only a word, but that life is real."

Karen
Age 17

Foreword

THE TERM *learning disability,* as well as all of its attendant behaviors, has become an acceptable and legitimate phrase in the dictionary of educational jargon. Rarely does one open an educational journal without finding some reference to learning disabilities. In these periodicals and in texts we find lists of materials, behaviors and symptoms, and unusual techniques for "curing" learning disabilities. We find esoteric studies and advertisements for, or discussions of, some fancy new test or remedial and/or diagnostic kits. We hear about the new, the newer, and the newest theories of learning disabilities. Professionals have quickly jumped on one bandwagon or another. They argue about which theoretical school has the answers. In a meeting of ten or twenty or thirty of these knowledgeable people one could find members of one or more of the following schools of thought: the endogenous, the exogenous, the biochemical, the psychoanalytic, the behavioral, the neurophysiological, the medical model, the neuropsychological, the developmental, the environmental, the linguistic, the psycholinguistic, the humanistic, and even the theological. And the discussions go on and on . . .

However, for the past twenty-seven years there has been one man who has not involved himself in these meaningless discussions. He has dedicated his professional life to teaching, interacting, and helping learning-disabled children overcome their learning difficulties. Dr. Donald E. Lyman has witnessed every major trend and fad that has been presented to the teaching profession. He has not participated in any bandwagon mania, but, in his own quiet way, he has been very involved in setting the pace for us to recognize and help children with learning problems. His experiences are real and his successes are fact.

I have worked with Don Lyman for over fifteen years, utilizing his proven methods in my university teaching and while I served as Director of the Newell C. Kephart Memorial Child Study Center at the University of Northern Colorado. I have included many of Don's ideas in well over a dozen of my published articles and presentations at national conferences in Georgia, Florida, Colorado, Michigan, and Illinois. In the early seventies I designed a teacher-training program in learning disabilities at Florida Atlantic University with several components based upon my observation of Don Lyman's work with children. In addition, over the past eight years I have witnessed the implementation of his program with hundreds of children at Troywood School in West Palm Beach, Florida.

It is difficult to identify the single most important aspect of Don's contribution to the field. Perhaps it is the fact that many years ago Don was one of the first to realize that learning-disabled children are concrete, creative, and nonsemantic thinkers. Therefore, we must consider these learning *abilities* in the presentation of academic material so that steady and continuous learning can occur. However, the key to Don's work is most probably the fact that he is one of the very few educators who emphasize the many positive qualities of learning-disabled children. I remember a comment he made some years back. "These children," he said, "are quite unusual. At one moment they are imaginative, if frivolous, observers of objects, interested in enjoying something as it is and moving to the next thing. At the next moment, they are interested in the parts and pieces of objects, breaking them down, building them up. Seeing how they relate. This is a rare combination of qualities. Most of us are one way or the other. Culture expects that there will be artists and mechanics, but not artistic-mechanics."

It is interesting that almost every new theory in the field has been predicated upon the assumption that the learning-disabled are disabled and have weaknesses. With this in mind, educators have either concentrated their efforts in remediating these weaknesses or totally forgetting about them and focusing on the learning strengths. Don Lyman has consistently told professionals and parents that we are talking about, first and foremost, a child with learning strengths and then learning weaknesses. His programs are specifically designed with such vision that we can build upon a child's positive qualities, teach him through his strengths, and at the same time help to remediate his academic skill and process weaknesses.

In his unique programs Don Lyman has demonstrated that we can blend remediation and compensation in developing both process and academic skill areas. I do hope that you will read this book with the same enthusiasm and understanding and hope for the future as I had. I am most pleased that Don has chosen to share his successes with us, and as a result of reading his book I am convinced that learning disabilities can be overcome.

Robert S. Sloat
Professor Emeritus
Human Rehabilitative Service
University of Northern Colorado

Part One

Prelude: Where I'm Coming From

Memories of Struggle

JEREMY'S STOMACH DOESN'T HURT TODAY. His eyes aren't wet. His mouth isn't tremulous; his face isn't smudgy. His fingertips, at rest now, look as if they might someday, somehow, recover from the relentless long-term shredding they have suffered. His chunky frame, overstretched by nervous eating, looks unnatural, incidental, able to reverse itself.

Jeremy found out today that he could read, like almost everybody else. He was seeing letters instead of cluttered, meaningless designs. He was hearing sounds inside his head that assembled into real words instead of gibberish.

Today faking is unnecessary; waiting for teacher to give clues is not required; stretching the memory in a way it refuses to stretch is needless. In fact, stomachaches, crying, finger biting, and faking have been options discarded by Jeremy for several months now.

"Boy, am I reading good today," Jeremy tells me, without turning his nose from the book. Not a question, not a probe, but a frank, hearty, uncalculated statement.

"You bet you are," I replied. Jeremy stops reading, turns his nose and eyes from the book and points them at me.

"Why couldn't I read before? Why was I dumb before?"

"You were never dumb, Jeremy. And you couldn't read before because letters and sounds for letters didn't make sense to you."

"Why do they make sense now?"

"Because now your brain not only knows all the things around you, but it can give those things names. Names that you can see and read."

Jeremy keeps probing. "Why couldn't it do that before?"

"Maybe it wasn't interested enough."

"That's not so. I always wanted to read."

"But your brain didn't. It was more interested in the real bike you rode than the letters b-i-k-e. More interested in the food you ate than f-o-o-d. But you have it trained now to know words as well as real things."

"Thanks for training my brain, Mr. Lyman."

"You did the training, Jeremy."

"Yahoo," says Jeremy, flipping his eyes upward in an attempt to stare at his brain. "I'm in charge now, brain, and you'd better do what I want or I'll knock your brains out." Jeremy almost falls out of his seat laughing at himself.

"That's stupid. That's a lot of crap."

This critique comes from Caroline, seated two seats to the left of Jeremy. Good old "Choleric Caroline." She can always be counted on to counter any human foible with the zing of a viper.

"That wasn't necessary," I tell Caroline, though I knew that for Caroline it was quite necessary.

"He's a real pinhead," says Caroline. "Just because he thinks he can read now, he's gotta brag and make up stupid jokes and not let me concentrate. If he wants a knock on his small brain, I'll give it to him."

Now Caroline is small, slender, and feminine looking. A poodle in appearance with the temperament and jaws of a pit bull.

"Caroline," I say, "sweet Caroline, Jeremy's happy because he can read better now than he could before. Why don't you try to be happy with him?"

"I'll be happy when he shuts his yap. And if he doesn't, I'll be happy when I shut it for him."

"Shut up!" This comes from Jeremy. Not a very creative or forceful effort, but his brain was absorbed in reading.

"You fat, weird pig. You used to cry. Now you flap your snout. Watch out, you blob. You're asking to be mashed like the potato you are." Caroline's vocabulary is concrete, rambling, and effective.

"Caroline," I say, "sweet Caroline. You're not angry at Jeremy. You're angry at yourself."

"Yeah, I am mad at me. I try to learn this stuff you give me to do and I can't learn it. It's so stupid. School's so stupid. You're stupid for trying to make me do this stuff. My mom's stupid because she thinks I'm stupid. My dad's stupid because he says everything will be all right and I know it won't. My brother's stupid even though he's good in school. He's stupid because he calls me retarded. Pretty soon, I'm not going to be able to handle all of this stupidness. I'm going to run away from this stupid world I'm in and go somewhere where I can be stupid all by myself without all this crappy stupidness all around me."

I say to Caroline, "Stupid is your favorite word."

"You're right," she answers. "I'm stupid. Everybody's stupid. Stupid, stupid, stupid, stupid, stupid, stupid." Then she cries and I thank God that Jeremy doesn't try to console her.

I rejoice with Jeremy and I grieve with Caroline. I am positive that Jeremy will flourish. I would be surprised if Caroline doesn't. But she mustn't quit on herself. I grieve with this bright child because she suffers an unjust anguish inflicted by a system that should have understood her better, tendered her more inspired teaching, and let her keep her ability to wonder. It is for the sake of every Jeremy and every Caroline that I tell my story and write whatever else is in this book.

I was born in a small upstate New York town in 1935. I don't know if I was born "learning disabled" or developed it later. In fact, when I became aware enough to realize that I had certain problems, I had no label like Specific Learning Disability to categorize them, so I thought that I was the only one in the world who had them. I don't know if I became aware of the problem before I started school, but I doubt it. First of all, I have very few recollections of preschool happenings and feelings, and second, there existed in pre–World War II days little searching out of preschool "signs" that might later lead to learning problems, or awareness that such signs existed.

Once I entered school, however, I became acutely aware that what I was expected to learn would not be easy. I was enrolled in a parochial school and found kindergarten fun most of the time. We played all day and I was a great player. I do remember one embarrassing incident though. One day Sister managed to get together a bunch of play horns and drums and arranged for all of us kindergarteners to make a daily parade around the block like a marching band. (If you remember, parades were very "in" during the early 1940s.) I was given a drum and expected to have some rhythm. I didn't. Sister tried to teach me a simple "boom" with the left hand, "ta, ta" with the right hand, and "boom" again with the left. I couldn't learn it. It came out "boom, boom, ta" or "boom, ta, boom, ta"; when I tried to repeat the sequence, I was in even deeper trouble, for I would hit two "booms" or two "ta's" with the left hand and throw the whole parade off cadence. Sister was very kind in retrospect. She didn't label me S.L.D. (slow-learning drummer); she simply decided that the band would have one "boom, boom" man — and I became great in that role. We marched around the block day after day with the horns blaring and all the drummers drumming "boom" (left hand), "ta, ta" (right hand), "boom" (left hand), except me. I was in the back going "boom, boom, pause, boom, boom, pause," all with my right hand. I became very successful at this and enjoyed the attention it brought me. Yet I do remember sitting at home wondering why I couldn't do "boom, ta, ta, boom" when everyone else could. Either they were smarter than I was or they practiced alone where nobody could see them. I was going to practice alone too, but I decided that the "boom, ta, ta, boom" people in the world far outnumbered "boom, boom" people. I decided to forget the practice and maintain my unique status as the only "boom, boom" person in the parade.

When I graduated into the world of "readin', 'ritin', and 'rithmetic," circumstances became tougher and rationalizing more difficult. I wasn't sure if *d* was itself or *p, g,* or *b*; or if *b* was *p, g,* or *d*; or if *q* was *p, d,* or *b*; or if *p* was *d, b,* or *g*; *h* and *n* and *6* and *9* gave me a hassle too. Once I remember the word *hen* came up in my reader and I read "you." Sister said, "What?" And I said, "You" and spelled it out loud for emphasis. "Y-e-u," I spelled. Everybody laughed. "Boom-Boom" was losing status fast.

Sometimes I wasn't sure which side of a word to start at; sometimes I wasn't sure which side of the page to start at. Recently I was going through some old books in my mother's attic. I came upon a yellowed sheet of paper with my name, St. John's School, Grade Two, and AMḊG on top of the page. AMḊG are the Latin initials for, "To the greater glory of God." What followed couldn't have glorified God very much. The first written line read, "The brid flwe over the huoes." There were other lines similar to this. There also was an F just below AMḊG.

I remember many other things that confused me. Those typewritten *a*'s looked so strange to me that I was never sure which letter I was dealing with. I was always saying "how" for *who* or the other way around. I don't know why it happened but I sometimes mixed up *y* and *v*. Everybody laughed when I read that Tom went out to play in the vard. I could usually tell a *6* from a *9*, but I had to concentrate on whether the vertical line was straight or not because I wasn't sure if up was down or which side was which. The *2* used to anger me because it looked a lot like **a**, and I felt very stupid when I confused a letter with a number. I knew that reading started at one side and math (after it got hard) started at the other, but I was never sure which side was which. I remember one day that another student said "saw" for *was*. I thought it was *saw* too, but since everyone laughed as usual, I pretended it was *was*. Sometime later I said "same" for *was*. I even think I remember seeing an *e* on the end of the word, but nobody else did. In this instance, the teacher was not so kind. She corrected the hecklers with something like this: "It's not funny. God did not make all of us smart." Boom-Boom's days of glory were only a memory. I remember thinking that as one gets older, he can't transfer the glory of his "boom-boom" days to the *was, saw, same* days of maturity. Looking back, letters and numbers were as arbitrary to me as the division between heaven and hell taught at my school. And I was in hell. Perhaps this is why some of my recollections from this period are so vivid.

But I developed an intense determination to turn school into a nice place for me. I could have chosen to escape. Three escape routes were open to me. I could have become a clown, diverting attention from my difficulty to my "funny" personality. I can remember James C., who did this successfully. He clowned his way from third grade through eighth grade and then dropped out of school. He had terrible grades, but his tactic worked. Everybody thought of James as funny, not stupid. So he escaped from school with an intact self-image and was able to clown his way eventually into becoming a super salesman. Today he owns an insurance agency. I did not choose this route because I didn't think I was a funny person and I knew I had no chance of competing with James.

Another escape open to me was the delinquency route. I could have started to skip school, break windows, get into fights, and cause trouble any way I could imagine, always stopping just short of getting into real trouble with the police.

Adults would think I was bad, kids would think I was tough and fearless; nobody would think I was stupid. Marty D. chose this route. I know that he was having the kind of difficulty in learning school work that I was having. He saw *p* for *b* sometimes, and *was* for *saw.* I admired Marty greatly and feared him so I remember a number of things that he did. Once he had to read, "What is your name?" and he read, "What is your man?" Nobody laughed at Marty, not if he wanted to survive recess. I didn't go to the same high school as Marty, but I learned that he earned a long suspension from school midway through tenth grade and never went back. I couldn't possibly have followed Marty's route; I was too "chicken." Marty owns and operates a successful construction company today.

Charlie J. chose the final escape route. Charlie went along with Sister's proclamation that God did not make us all smart. Charlie actually chose to be stupid. Everybody felt sorry for him and tried to help him. Even though Charlie was a big, rugged guy, he became the class pet. "Poor Charlie," Sister and the kids would say with a look of pity and affection etched in their eyes. I could never, never have chosen Charlie's route, even though I knew he had the same trouble that I had. I think I would have jumped off the school roof before submitting to "Poor Don" and pitiful, affectionate looks. Apparently, Charlie was just playing a "survival" game in school, for his self-image also remained intact. He dropped out of school after eighth grade graduation and probably never heard another "Poor Charlie." That very summer he got a job pumping gas, which we all admired. Today he owns five service stations.

As I said, I chose none of these routes. The only way out that I could conceive was to engage in the tremendous struggle to become "normal." Had I been given an acceptable label like Specific Learning Disability to identify my problem, I think I would have been glad to have it pinned on me. I can't speak for James or Marty or Charlie, but I suspect that they would have embraced the label along with me. If this had happened, I wonder what the four of us would be doing today. But doctors, educators, psychologists, and parents did not perceive it within their scope back then to encapsulate us in the comforting cocoon of Specific Learning Disability, so James, Marty, and Charlie chose their routes and I chose to become a normal student at any cost.

In a sense I withdrew. I kept a few close friends and spent some time with them, but most of the time I spent alone, studying. I passed long hours tracing and retracing letters, words, and numbers so that I could develop some degree of assurance that I was seeing them the way almost everybody else did. I remember reading and rereading passages in my school books until I had them memorized. Then I would ask myself questions about their content. I do not have clear recollection of many of the means I used to train myself, but I'm sure that many of the procedures I describe in this book stem from fragmented recollections of my early years.

My hours of self-training paid off. I was able to keep up with my class. Eventually I became an excellent student, but not without a continuing struggle.

The transition to cursive writing was especially difficult for me. I couldn't easily see the difference between *oa* and *ou* or *au* and *ao* or *ao* and *oo*; or *va*, *vo*, and *vu*. Consonants as well as vowels caused me trouble. I mixed up *n* and *m* and *M* and *N*; *b*, *g*, and *d* continued to confuse me, and somehow I found a way to reverse them regularly, even in cursive writing. I remember having great difficulty crossing *t*'s with a horizontal line. They always ended up looking like this: " 𝘟 " or like this: " 𝘵 ." No matter how often the teacher circled them in red, I still couldn't correct them. I really couldn't see how they were wrong. True to my pattern, I tied myself down to seemingly endless practice sessions, tracing and retracing, writing and rewriting, practicing letters in every combination I could think of, doing assignments requiring cursive writing ten times both for the practice and to make sure that my copy for the teacher was presentable. My father used to chase me out of the house. "Don't stay cooped up," he would say. "Go make friends." Eventually I became proficient in cursive writing, and to my surprise this proficiency improved my spelling and my reading fluency. I know now why this happened and will explain later in this book. But back then it was pure serendipity.

I have two other recollections from my years in elementary school. One is extracurricular and the other goes to the very core of my early school experience.

BB guns were very popular when I was in elementary school. Every boy I knew had his Red Ryder and I had mine too. Where I lived, there were plenty of woods within walking distance of everybody's home, and people didn't mind kids using BB guns as much as they do now. I remember my Red Ryder causing me constant embarrassment, even nightmares. It seemed that I could never bring that gun to the same shoulder twice in a row. I would attempt to aim with my left eye only to find that that was the one I closed. I'd switch over to the right eye and inadvertently close it while thinking that I was keeping it open. When I became furious enough, I would hold the gun in the middle at the ridge of my nose and try to aim with both eyes open. As I think back now, I can feel the hard bumps that my Red Ryder inflicted on my nose. I can also remember my friends heckling me. My aim was so erratic that I became known as "The Lone Danger."

I also remember from the elementary years (fifth or sixth grade, I think) that we were given IQ tests. The teachers explained beforehand that the tests were designed to show how well we could think. I panicked instantly and without reservation. Wild thoughts ran through my mind. Sure, I got passing grades most of the time, but I was really very stupid because nobody else had to study as hard as I did. Now my secret "problem in stupidity" was going to be discovered. Thank God that we weren't forewarned about the tests a week in advance. I would have worried myself into a severe neurosis. Here was a test that I couldn't study for, couldn't prepare for. The image of myself as a normal student and human being that I had labored so hard to build for so many hours of so many days was going to be shattered.

As it turned out, the teacher put the test in front of us immediately after explaining its purpose. My initial panic carried over into the test. I could hardly read it. Letters, numbers, and words hardly looked the same twice in a row. When I finally figured out the words in a question, I forgot their meaning. When I finally got the meaning of each word in the question and started to put together the meaning of the whole question, I would forget the meaning of the individual words again. I ended up guessing at most answers.

A few days after completion of the test (days filled with fear and depression) my worst fear was confirmed. I spied a list of the test results on the teacher's desk and my name was near the bottom of the list. Only James, Marty, and Charlie were below me, but they didn't pretend to be smart as I did. I thanked God daily that the teacher didn't read the results to the class or post the list. For weeks I dreaded facing each school day for fear that she might do one of these two things. Even after this fear subsided, I could not look the teacher in the eye for the rest of the school year. (She was the one who made the list and knew I was stupid — no covering up with her.) I wasn't as comfortable as before with the other students either. Maybe some of them saw the list on the desk, just as I did. One thing is for sure. Buried somewhere in some file cabinet, locked for years, is the school record of a fourth grader with a 72 IQ — a fourth grader who some years later was Phi Beta Kappa.

Still, with the one exception of the IQ test, I continued to build success upon success in school. I think I was trying to prove to myself and everybody else that I wasn't stupid. I became a professional student. Every weekday evening and a large chunk of every weekend was dedicated to study. I learned to memorize whole pages and practiced writing them from memory. I was so overprepared for tests that it seemed as if I had the textbook glued in my mind when I took them. If I couldn't figure out an answer, I'd simply replay the text in my mind until the answer appeared. When a new kind of problem came up in math, I would do every similar problem in the text and worksheets many times over, until the method became as familiar to me as walking. I wrote out everything many times because I learned more easily and remembered better that way.

By the time I reached my junior year in high school, it was rare that I didn't achieve an A in all subjects. If there is such a creature as an "overachiever," I was one. Some educators and some parents still worry about "overachievement." I would urge you not to waste your worry. Overachievement accompanied by hard academic self-discipline builds self-concept; it doesn't destroy it.

In college I decided to become a history major and teach history. History was easy for me because it required much memorizing, and I had trained my memory well. I also enjoyed associating ideas and events and dreaming up novel ways of arranging them and drawing conclusions. So I did very well. I was elected to the National Social Science Honor Society and graduated Phi Beta Kappa. But I didn't become a history teacher; there were too many history teachers around. I had to settle for an elementary school teaching position in New York City. The year was 1956. The day after Labor Day I walked into a room filled almost to bursting with forty-nine fifth graders. Before the first week was finished, I learned that at least fifteen of these children were having the same difficulty that I had. At first, viewing the situation from my side of the desk, I didn't like those fifteen children at all. They weren't like I used to be. They didn't spend three or four hours every day trying to catch up to their "normal" class-mates and surpass them. They seemed dedicated to the prop-osition that they were stupid and that stupid students were put on this earth to give teachers (especially new teachers) a hard time. I was launching a new career and wanted to suc-ceed with the same determination that had made me succeed in school. This "mean fifteen" caused me continuous stress. Success no longer meant disciplining myself but disciplining them. The task seemed impossible. How could life have dealt me this dirty hand? Why spend all of your life fighting to be "normal" and then be threatened by your mirror image? I was ready to quit. I would have quit in an instant if somebody had offered me another way to eat. Nobody did, so I kept up the struggle. When Tom refused to read because he had read the same story last year; when Jeff missed 23 out of 25 words on a spelling test and told me it was my fault because I "talked funny"; when Juan insisted that 17 + 28 was 315 and I was stupid for saying otherwise because his father taught him how to do it and his father would be glad to come over

and punch some sense into me; when Frank made a $\mathcal{f}$ and

insisted it was a *j*, *f*, *p*, *q*, *E*, *G*, *S*, *T*, or *L*, depending on the circumstances; when Larry declared that ½ of a pound was less than ¹⁄₁₆ of a pound because his teacher had taught him that last year — and where did I learn how to teach anyhow; when these unlabeled learning-disabled kids messed up every attempt I made at teaching the regular kids (and, worst of all, the "regulars" loved them and sought to imitate them), I nearly cried inside. I gave all my life to overcoming my own "Dumbo" self-image and here I was having my new self-image deflated daily by a new crop of "Dumbos."

I wish I could say that some dramatic incident or insight

brought me "to the light," but this didn't happen. I simply decided one day to conquer the "mean fifteen" or quit teaching and become whatever a dropout teacher becomes. I think my many years of solitary, disciplined study hardened me for this struggle. After deciding to fight — I fought. Nothing can be more draining than to give constant attention to a side show when the main event is more attractive. (I loved my "regulars"; after all, I struggled many years to become one.) But I realized that I would never be able to teach them anything until I subdued the "mean fifteen." So I diverted my attention to them, not because I felt empathy toward them but because I was tired of their interference with my efforts to be a good teacher. I was determined that the "mean fifteen" would be as "regular" as the other students were and as "regular" as I had become.

It really came as no surprise to me when I found that I was able to "see into" the perceptions, thoughts, and feelings of these children. The experience was like a playback of similar perceptions, thoughts, and feelings that had been imprinted on my mind years before. I worked earnestly to "normalize" these children, and they began to change. They didn't become conventional students in a week or a month or even by year's end. But they began to try and began to succeed. Many small day-after-day successes merged and pyramided into self-assurance.

Juan typified the mean fifteen's willingness and ability to change. He was a dual dyslexic, unable to read, spell, or write in two languages. For Juan, Spanish at home and English in school were meant for speaking purposes only and Juan delighted in using them for this purpose. He spoke and spoke and spoke. I don't imply here that he had a large vocabulary. On the contrary, his vocabulary was extraordinarily limited and extremely moderate in scope. (At least in school.) Juan earned his garrulous reputation by using the same twenty-five to thirty words to punctuate every event, describe every feeling, and solve every problem, abstract or concrete, human or mechanical. Let me give you a sampling of "Juan's words." I make an epithet out of this because the phrase "Juan's words" was to become a class byword.

You'll notice that a few Spanish words are mixed in. Juan tried to keep his Spanish words at home for "esocial reasons" as his father would have it, but the same few always slipped out at school. Here, for your reading gratification, are "Juan's words":

> Smash, break, punch, kill, ponche, bleed, blood, hurt, golpe, tough, chicken, stab, kick, scratch, knock [in every direction — up, off, down, in, out], crack, split, crush, gusano, tear, fight, hack, wound, bruise, wipe out, spoil, slit, rip, gangster, tortura, and sorry.

A few comments on "Juan's words." First, I censored some of his words for school purposes. These words do not appear in the above list either. Second, Juan knew the names of every body part in addition to the above words, for he usually threatened to do most of the above to one or the other of them. Third, Juan used *sorry* more than any other word because he seldom meant what he said. Choosing words from his own vocabulary, I can say without hesitation that he was a "wounded chicken" and his words were a wall to hide behind.

Back to my efforts to normalize the mean fifteen. I felt sure that they would never be able to perceive words efficiently or remember them until they could "image" them (see them in their minds). So I initiated a daily procedure of standing in the back of the room, insisting that all students keep heads forward and eyes closed. When I had set this scene (a more difficult task than you can imagine), I spelled a word, snapped my fingers and expected my students to say the word after the snap. In this way, I hoped the students would "image" each letter in sequence and retain all of them long enough to recognize the word. This procedure seemed to work as planned for the regulars, but the mean fifteen were not imaging. They were echoing the regulars. I wanted to take the mean fifteen into another room and drill the procedure into them starting with the simplest words, but I had nobody to entertain the regulars. For this reason, I divided the class into two uneven parts, the regulars and the fifteen. With the former, I used appropriate words from the basal reading series. With the fifteen, I used "Juan's words."

Starting with the fifteen, I spelled "s-m-a-s-h." Furrowed brows, bent heads, scratched scalps, but not a sound.

"S-m-a-s-h," I spelled again — and again and again, finally blending letter name and sound to the point that I was almost saying the word.

"Ess-em-aah-ess-sha."

"Cow," shouted Tom.

"Tree," suggested Frank.

"United States," said Larry with great dignity.

"Gusanos," sneered Juan at the rest of the fifteen. At me, he turned his head, opened his eyes, smiled broadly, and said, "Scratch."

"No," I said. "But you're close. You got the s at the beginning, the a in the middle, and the h at the end."

"Shitword," cursed Juan. "Knock off my ears. They're no good. They're cracked."

"Don't snap at your friends or your ears."

"Sorry," said Juan.

"And don't be sorry that you're wrong. You came close."

"Sorry," said Juan.

"And don't turn your head."

"Sorry."

"And keep your eyes closed."

"Sorry."

"And try to see every letter inside your head before you make a stab at it."

"Stab the word. That's good. Stab the word. Oops. Sorry."

"*Ess-em-aah-ess-shu, s-m-a-s-h,*" *I spelled.*

"*Smash,*" *shouted Juan.* "*I smash your head. I smash your face. I smash the wall. I don't stab the word. I smash it. Oops. Sorry, Mr. Lyman.*"

"*Good, Juan, you got it.*"

"*Sorry.*"

"*Don't be sorry. You got it.*"

"*Oh, tough. I wiped it out. I knocked it down. I killed it.*"

"*Yes, you did.*"

It wasn't very long before the rest of the mean fifteen were recognizing "Juan's words" by letter names only.

The regulars became rebellious. They were tiring of words like *beseech, adduce, console, abundant,* and *flexible.* They preferred Juan's concrete vocabulary. Every day I heard more of "We want 'Juan's words.' Why can't we have 'Juan's words'? How come *they* get 'Juan's words' and we don't?"

So I gave everybody "Juan's words." At first, singly, then in phrase, sentence, and finally in paragraph form. Eventually, all the class (even the mean fifteen) were writing paragraphs with "Juan's words."

Juan, of course, prospered with this overkill of attention and soon became too good for his own vocabulary. I remember one of his paragraphs well enough to reconstruct it:

> I will smash anybody who punches or makes peopul bleed. I will knock there teath in. They are gusanos and I will fight them. I will wipe them out and hert them. Sorry I hab to do this. I am a goob man. God Blast you. Thes is form my hart. Lob to eberyboby. Sorry.
>
> Juan

Juan became so motivated to read and to write that the other members of the mean fifteen could hardly resist his charisma augmented by his threats to "crush your brain if you don't try. Sorry."

I carry guilt from my first year's teaching. I didn't teach the regulars much. I rationalize my guilt in three ways:

1. The regulars would have learned without me.
2. I entertained them a lot with a big boost from the mean fifteen.
3. You can't be all things to all people. Sorry.

I began to enjoy what I was doing and gradually came to the realization that life had dealt me a better hand than I thought. Up to this day (twenty-seven years later), I have been working daily with learning-disabled children and have found them clever, fascinating, enjoyable people. God even blessed me with one learning-disabled child out of four of my own. (Since I was spending my life in the learning-disability business, He must have felt that my family should be an approximate example of the national average.)

Before the SLD (Specific Learning Disability) label came into vogue, I requested and was gladly given the lowest groups on the homogeneous ladder wherever I taught. By today's standards, these groups were seventy-five percent learning disabled. The only difference was the number of students in the groups — thirty-five to forty instead of the customary eight to twelve in today's SLD units. By 1964, labels and handicaps and syndromes had become acceptable and respectable, so I went back to school to become certified in the new field of Specific Learning Disability. Since that time I have taken almost every course available in this field, as well as in Emotional Handicap. I continue to acquaint myself with any new course or program that promises to give me new insights and techniques.

I stand against some recent trends I have observed. Some teacher education courses, professional journals, and SLD organizations have been giving much emphasis to compensation, coping, and handicap adjustment. I sometimes find my profession telling me to teach compensatory and adjustment skills, while my experience tells me that I can teach learning-disabled children to overcome or, at least, to master their handicap. It also tells me that the SLD syndrome is real. I cannot join those who would call it a myth or a fabrication to excuse parental guilt feelings or to market drugs to children. But I cannot be comfortable with those who teach only coping, compensating, and adjusting. If I can teach *one* learning-disabled child to overcome his handicap, then the handicap can be overcome. I have taught hundreds (including myself) how to overcome specific learning disability and function with success and confidence (not merely cope) in a variety of academic, social, and occupational settings.

2

Memories Without Words, Followed by Head Noise

MILLIONS OF CHILDREN are experiencing today what I experienced four decades ago. As I mentioned earlier, this book is written on behalf of these children. In this book, I attempt to make some sense out of (or put some sense into) their confounding experiences with language, learning, and even life, for life intersects language and learning at so very many of its moments.

I felt that my personal childhood experience should be a part of this book. For this reason, it became necessary to shift my memory into the long term and engage it in recollecting experiences of my early school days or daze (take your choice — both words are appropriate). As a result of this effort, recollections came to me in a jumble of words that spoke of action, struggle, failure, anxiety, and victory. These recollections are described in chapter 1.

Occasionally, however, memories of a very different sort emerged, but only, it seemed, when I was not trying to remember. These memories were not a matter of words. They pictured a child who lived at least part time in a world without words and other symbols. For some, thinking in words is the only human kind of thinking. I wonder about that.

My memories unveiled a child who spent long periods of

time engaged in thoughtful action, seldom thinking a single word. Let me suggest that you let your memory wander back to your own childhood. Picture yourself as a child without trying to remember any particular instance. Perhaps you will be rewarded with images similar to mine.

I played marbles often, occasionally most of a weekend. Like many of my friends, I took pride in my marble collection without thinking, "I am proud of this collection." I marveled at the beauty and variety of their colors without thinking, "This one is blue and white. This one is orange, yellow, and black." I regretted losing a favorite to an opponent without thinking, "There goes a favorite." The thought (without words) always came first and was abstracted into words only when I wanted to communicate it. I plotted the most subtle game strategies, calculated complicated vectors and angles of trajectory, second-guessed my opponents, estimated velocity, and examined surfaces for ruts and obstacles without thinking a single letter, word, or number.

Other weekends were spent building tree forts. My father liked carpentry, so tools, nails, and wood remnants in many shapes and sizes were usually available. Forts were assembled, disassembled, moved to better spots, and reassembled. Unmatchable wood remnants were matched or nearly matched before being nailed and patched afterward. Sometimes pieces were overlapped to support each other, for nails usually ran out and who wanted to go all the way back to the house for more. The building crew would run to the fort whenever it rained to "test it out," and leaks would mandate instant repair or reconstruction after the storm. What a strong visual, tactile, aural, carefree, "good ole me and my friends" image I get now as I write this. New blond wood and old gray-brown wood nailed together in happy integration; wind whistling through cracks, rain hammering the fort almost as loudly as the hammer that had driven in its nails only hours before. Reach out and touch the wood, the bent nails.

Fingers asking, "Why didn't that one go straight?" And me sitting there, feeling safe and self-fulfilled in a structure artfully engineered by me. There are no words in this image. In fact, almost all of the human thought and energy that went into the fort's construction were expended without the intervention of words, either inside the head or without. Words were conjured up only to praise or vilify the products of thought.

"Hey, not a drop of rain [or a ray of sunlight] can get in!"
"You moron, you forgot the window [or door]!"

or

"Look, the rain's getting in only through your section. [Section. What's a section? Where'd that word come from? Oh well.] Your sek shon, Johnny, your sek shon, the sek shon you made, stinks."

I recall another absorbing pastime, enjoyed most of the time alone. I was lucky to have a very large wooded area, at least a few miles deep, within a block of home. At the farthest northeast corner was a high fence that marked the outmost boundary of a state prison. I recall starting at various points along the perimeter of the woods and exploring different routes to the fence, trying to plot the most direct route from each starting point. When a sufficient number of direct routes had been established to satisfy me, I plotted my way to the fence, searching out other routes — the most dangerous, the most scenic, or the most gentle routes (ones that my little brother could follow). I mapped these routes on paper and delighted in their intersections. Here's a gentle spot on a dangerous route, or a scenic spot on the direct route, or a dangerous, scenic, gentle spot. How is that possible? Back into the woods to check that one out.

One day I was Lewis; the next day, Clark; the next day, Livingston-I-presume; Coronado, the next; De Soto, the next; and a great, nameless Indian pathfinder, the next. I enjoyed being the Indian most because I fancied I was swift, stealthy, quiet, instinctive, and fearless, needing help from no man. Sometimes I imagined myself a mythical god of sorts or a great old-fashioned saint or a medieval wizard who could cause the woods to do my bidding and the sky to change at my whim and the shifty creatures of the forest to lend me their wordless thoughts. But too often words would find their way into my brain, and hidden among those words was the most awful word of all — *school*. And I would think "school" and run home to watch the clock, because Monday came slower that way and it came so fast in the woods.

Doubtless, all of this is but a sampling of the commonplace childhood imagination and magic that most of us experienced as half-pints. I experienced most of it, I am certain (like Jeremy and Caroline, and Juan and Frank and Larry and . . .), without thinking in words, without naming, defining, or mulling over my every objective, action, or state of being, without the distraction of continuous brain chatter. And I suspect that some of you may have experienced it in a similar way.

How then did I (and perhaps you) experience the fantasy of childhood? More often than not, I am sure, in very concrete and basically real terms. Just as the thirsty horse goes for the water trough without thinking, "I'm going to go over there for a drink"; just as the falcon flies for the highest perch in sight without thinking, "What's a perch? And where is the highest? And why am I flying there? And just what is flying, anyway?"; just as a dog lies secure at the feet of the master without thinking, "I'm guaranteed food here, but this is a hell of a way to spend a Saturday night"; and just as a human can experience an event deeply (beyond the heart, into the gut, transcending even that), an event that words can't express, that maybe tears or laughter or shrugs or complacency or love can, so I lived part time as a child and so, possibly, did you.

But how did I think? How did I perform? Was I acting less

human, more animal, when I acted without words in my head? Did I reach human status only when my mind became totally oriented to words and could hardly function without them?

Let me answer one question at a time. I thought, to the best of my recollection, in strong visual images. Quite simply, I pictured in my mind what I had just done and what I planned to do next. What I was doing, I simply did. A kind of sensory motor intelligence, a "body knowing," guided me. You have experienced a similar knowing when you served a tennis ball, typed a letter, diapered a baby, or danced the night away. We all know that directing such activities with words causes a sudden sharp drop in performance.

My visual images were often combined with sounds. Not surprising, because most visible objects and actions make noises. The images were also preceded or accompanied by impressions or feelings that monitored their appropriateness. It was a kind of jaunty thinking and feeling that dealt only in concrete reality and enabled me to embrace life with enthusiasm. I did speak words and sentences in this nonsemantic world, but they were spontaneous expressions of feeling, unprepared and unedited comments, words more akin to gesture than to expression of logical thought. When I saw a grasshopper, for example, I did not think, "There goes a grasshopper" and let it go at that, allowing the symbol to substitute for the reality. I felt drawn (not in an introspective or conscious way) to look at the insect, examine it, listen to it, touch and feel it, if I could catch it. Later, if I thought of this experience, I did not think the words, "I saw a grasshopper" but rather I *imaged* the grasshopper, heard its sounds internally and felt its texture on my finger tips and inside them.

Consider an object as prosaic as a school desk. Even this was a real object to me rather than a "named" object. As I sat at it, I examined it constantly, feeling its lines and texture, scraping its varnish with fingernails, listening to its creaks and groans when I shifted position (desks were screwed to the floor back then), lifting its lid many more times than necessary to examine its innards and markings, circling its inkwell with my fingers, probing its nuts and bolts, carving its surface with pencil or pen to experience its density, filling its pencil slot with eraser bits, polishing it with elbow and examining the results. On a few occasions I even put my lips to the desk or sank my teeth into it. I'm sure the Sister considered this fairly bizarre behavior, and I'm grateful that she did not recommend me for psychiatric testing but limited her corrective measures to "Lyman, leave that desk alone."

I am certain that I spent my school hours engrossed in the reality of my desk rather than those fantasies of word manipulation called teaching and learning. Paradoxically, what I considered real, teachers considered fantasy. What I considered fantasy, they considered real. Words came at me like riddles, uninvited and boring. My desk happened to be there, inviting me to touch it and taste it.

In my wordless world, all that I encountered was real, for I encountered the concreteness of the object rather than its symbolic name. Even people were concrete to me. I remembered them better by their faces, gestures, gaits, clothing, eyes, expressions, colors, odors, and voices than by name. Even today I remember the faces, eyes, gaits, and scents of teachers that I liked, but I cannot recall their names.

My concrete world possessed many other qualities endearing to me in retrospect but hard to endure, I am sure, by those adults responsible for my maturation. Existence in my world followed no time line. Beginnings and endings were not important, for living and experiencing were spontaneous. I gave little significance to planning or prediction or control. I was not oriented toward goals, used little reflective memory, and had no future expectations. For these reasons I often left tasks unfinished or even forgotten, and I was late for scheduled activities more often than not.

I passed unmeasured amounts of time trying to put things together and make them work, or at least have the parts fit right — clocks, watches, engines, mechanical toys, appliances, furniture, puzzles, tools, and models. Sometimes I would disassemble working wholes just to have the opportunity to try to make them whole again. This penchant did not make me popular in my home or in friends' homes.

I passed even more time drawing. Not ordinary kid-type drawings like trees and houses and people, but extremely detailed drawings of wharves, docks, bridges, villages, house plans, battlefield scenes, the inner workings of complicated, imaginary machines, and lakes with hundreds of sailboats or oceans with thousands of battleships or a sky obliterated by huge fleets of bombers, fighter planes, and dirigibles. These drawings were not accompanied by brain chatter, naming parts and wholes and relationships as the drawings progressed. The only mind activity I recall, after the decision to draw, was an awareness of and delight in the spatial and directional patterns created and duplicated again and again by mind and hand.

My wordless world was also nonjudgmental and nonpersonal. I did not judge people or give importance to their judgments of me. Friends were those whose minds wandered and wondered with mine. They were not significant as people, only as sharers. There were no enemies, merely friends and not-friends.

I experienced a world without a need for hope or anticipation. Hope is futuristic. Since the present consumed me totally, hope had no place. Neither did fear or anxiety. I could be startled, no doubt, but I never feared because I never anticipated outcomes.

It is not surprising that my wordless memories are tinged with nostalgia. I have wondered often, after recalling this lost world, how I ever found the spunk to leave it in the first place and eventually abandon it altogether.

Now let me address the second question: Was I an imma-

ture human when I functioned without words? A developmental enigma that should have developed sooner? I don't
think so. My childhood affinity to the concrete realness of a
concrete world was, I am sure, an innate trait that all of us
possess to some degree. I had more of it than most. And I feel
that this very fact contributed to the difficulty that I had in
crossing the invisible boundary into the symbolic world — a
world of alphabets and reading and writing, of adding and
subtracting numbers instead of putting together and taking
apart real things. What sense did *b, d, u, n, m, w, p, q, s, z, t,*
+, −, ×, ÷ make to me? From the very first, I felt strange in
this world — uncomfortable, disoriented, homesick, threatened, and afraid. When it came to symbols (and in this world
it always did), my nerves were not suited, my eyes were not
adjusted, my ears were not tuned, my muscles were not fitted,
my brain was not receptive, and my mind was not interested.
This was my learning disability — an inability to make sense
of a representational world, a world in which an object as
named was more important than the object itself.

It is my opinion that bright, curious, itchy, overactive, annoying, immature, irresponsible children who can't read,
write, or do arithmetic well (our school-aged learning-disabled population) are concrete creatures caught up in a
wordy world, just as I was.

Speaking of words, I have a favorite one, for better or
worse. The word is *semantics*. It speaks of getting, feeling, re-
alizing meaning from symbols. This word defines the world
of words; it connotes (to me, at least) the peremptory character of that world and its haughtiness. People who can't cope
in that world are disabled. There are many, many children
(and adults, too) who can't manage to stay afloat on the semantic seas of this world, who are sinking daily in those seas
and not coming up. Recently, I heard a ten-year-old boy shout
in class, "Somebody help me. I'm in over my head." A few
months ago I was a guest on a TV talk show and proclaimed

that learning disability could be overcome. Many have written to me since then. A twenty-seven-year-old woman wrote, "There is no rescue for me and I don't have a job because of my disability. So I couldn't pay for help if I could find it." A fifty-seven-year-old man concluded his letter with the cry, "Help! Help!"

My recollections in chapter 1 speak of struggle, momentary failures, and ultimate victory. The victory, from one point of view, was a hard-earned, glorious triumph over a handicap that could have prevented my effective participation in a literate, semantic society. From another point of view, my victory was actually surrender. It was a very necessary surrendering *of* my concrete world and a very necessary surrendering *to* the semantic world of almost everybody else. On the time line of human history and evolution, I was an anachronism; my psychoneurological network did not seem updated enough to handle constant, rapid inputs of abstract symbols and semantics. It dysfunctioned under the pressure of these conditions, leaving me confused and groping. I remember teacher comments to this effect:

"Donald could not seem to function today."
"Donald seemed too confused or too shy to ask questions."
"If I slow down, Donald seems to do better."

As I mentioned in chapter 1, I decided to surrender to the pressures of normality mandated by the semantic culture I chanced into at birth. I realized, after starting my school life, that my stage and my script had already been prepared for me. I chose to become a good, even an excellent, actor. I wanted above all else to be normal or better than normal. Withdrawal into the comforts of my nonsemantic world was tempting, but I would not allow myself the comfort of "subnormality."

For this reason, at some forgotten interval between my tenth and eleventh birthdays, I plunged into the sea of semantics with the grittiness and drive of a channel swimmer. Then began a period of "head noise" that still echoes in my memory. Words filled my head and escaped my mouth continuously. Saying words, looking at words, subvocalizing words, thinking words, singing words, writing words, looking at and saying and writing words at the same time; saying and writing words without looking at them; eyes open — look at the words; eyes closed — write the words; always saying them, always thinking them; thinking them, saying them; writing them simultaneously, reading words, reading them from all angles, stretching sound symbols to accommodate writing speed, writing faster and speaking faster; graduating to sentences, graduating to paragraphs; memorizing sentences, memorizing paragraphs; reading them from memory, saying them from memory, writing them from memory; hundreds of words, thousands of words, tens of thousands of words, always in my head, making noise, noise that took on meaning, noise that made sense, semantic noise, during the school day, after school, at night, during night dreams and during day dreams.

Sooner than I thought possible, I was reading, spelling, and writing as well as most of my contemporaries. And most of this word learning I accomplished on my own. School provided the motivation, the impetus, the assignments, the testing ground, but not the life-controlling practice necessary to assimilate and imprint symbols and semantics into my dysfunctioning central nervous system.

The image I describe here — not the worried struggler, not the concrete thinker, but the successful overachiever — is the image I apparently projected to others.

A short while ago I asked a contemporary, a former teacher (now retired), and a few older family members and relatives, "What was Don Lyman like in school?" The answers I received were couched in kindness and were close to consensus. Here are two samples:

> "A slow starter, but a hard worker who usually did well."
> "A very hard worker. Had to study harder than most. Took school seriously."

As a result of the semantic monologues and semantic chatter that took up permanent residence in my mind-brain, I became an abstract thinker. Even when I engaged in concrete observations and experiences these monologues and that chatter prestructured the events and controlled my participation in them. My nonsemantic world disappeared without my awareness. In fact, it disappeared so completely that I lost awareness (until recently) that it had ever existed.

3

Mixed Emotions

I JOINED THE WORLD OF WORDS and forgot my world of marbles, tree forts, and trails. All of us had to make a similar move. We had to give up in order to get, bury our fundamental selves so that we could begin to grow into symbolic selves, while our parents and teachers and all the people responsible for our growth watered and waited.

I don't know your story, but I know that mine tells of a sacrifice that was total and supreme. There was no way that I could have entered the gate into the paradise of symbols, words, and abstract meanings without total commitment. It would have been easier for "a camel to go through the eye of a needle."

I did not become an immediate success in the symbolic world. I grew slowly, far more slowly than most of my contemporaries. I'm sure that the thought occurred to some of my peers and most of my teachers that I might not thrive in this soil. But I did thrive, and in the academic world of paper and mental puttering, I grew tall. In the seventh grade, I was struggling. By the ninth grade, I was holding my own. In the eleventh grade, I became a straight-A student. At my high school graduation, I was number two in my class. In college, I continued to grow. Almost every honor available was bestowed on me when I graduated. At the graduate school level, A's became as important to me as breathing, and almost as automatic.

How did I do it? How could a dyslexic (a reading- and writing-disabled person) become a scholar?

First, I had to relinquish any purpose in life other than learning to read, write, compute, and think with words. Other purposes had to be discarded as the distractions they truly were. In my case, this meant letting go of friends; staying indoors and using home as an insulation against the lure of outdoor life; curtailing leisure, fun, and sports; forbidding my mind to wander and especially not to wonder; losing sleep, spending a good part of each night forcing my mind to image the symbols of the day — this until my brain and body could take no more and shut themselves down; pretending to communicate with my family while my mind occupied itself with a constant stream of school-required symbols, sounds, and meanings unrelated to family concerns and pastimes; eating huge meals and not remembering taste or even what was eaten because my mind was dealing in symbols instead of enjoying food.

Second, I had to train myself to endure constant, emotion-numbing practice with symbols and semantics. Just as a marathoner has to "space out" in order to endure pain and achieve victory, so I had to space out of every concrete happening around me in order to endure the pain of practice and eventual success. I could not learn by simply reading something once or twice. I had to read it fifteen or twenty times and then write it as many times more. Then I had to say it and write it at the same time. After this, I had to be able to parrot it inside my head and image it there at the same time. If I couldn't do this, I had to go back to saying it and writing it again. If I still couldn't see and say it internally, I had to close my eyes, tighten my muscles, and swing my arms vigorously in the directions needed to re-create the letters of the words. In this way (almost by punching sense into my brain as a boxer gets the bag to do his bidding), I could finally mentally form the letters, words, and sentences. Even then, three problems remained: One, how to make sense out of words and sentences — the semantic problem. Two, how to complete long assignments when I had to spend hours just learning a short paragraph, maybe one twentieth of the assignment — the efficiency problem. Three, how to pretend that I knew what I was expected to know and didn't know while showing no sweat at all — the salvage-the-self-image problem.

I solved the semantic problem by pretending that I was in the situation described by the words — no matter that I might have to be a place or thing as well as a person — and acting out the situation. This usually worked well for me. Sometimes I would have to use one hand for a thing, another for a person, and my head, bobbing and swinging, as another person or something else. I showed action by movement and "just being" by staying still. These antics usually helped me to understand the message that the alphabet disguised.

I solved the efficiency problem (until I became more efficient) by learning only one small paragraph and ignoring the rest of the assignment.

I solved the self-image problem by acting alert and wisely passive while the assignment was being discussed by teacher and the rest of the class. There were always other students — many of them — eager to raise hands and volunteer answers. As you probably remember, teacher was always anxious to get a correct answer quickly so she called on the eager, hand-waving, beavers. I widened my eyes and nodded my head with approval when they were right; or wrinkled my eyes and wizened my brow with puzzlement when teacher declared them wrong. In the first instance, I hoped that teacher would assume that I, too, knew the answer if she happened to glance in my direction; in the second, I hoped that she would assume that I, too, was puzzled — wisely, of course — at the wrong answer. And, since she was sherlocking right answers, she would probably not call on me. Most of the time, I succeeded with this cover-up. When I did not, I flatly admitted (after many hours of studying) that I didn't have time to study.

"More important things came up, Sister."

"Like what?"

"Like watching my little brother, or weeding my dad's garden, or [for the benefit of my peers] tracking whatever animal is scaring my dad's chickens. He just built them a house so they could lay in peace and now this."

"And these activities were more important than your lessons?"

"Yes, Sister."

"WHAT!"

"I mean, 'No, Sister'; of course not." Good God, I had to call her sister but she was more like an angry stepmother than a sister.

"Nothing is more important than your lessons."

"Yes, Sister. I agree, Sister. Sorry, Sister."

And then followed a lecture on the ordering of priorities and I escaped again — irresponsible for sure, but not stupid.

When "my paragraph" came along, my moment in the sun, lies became unnecessary. I raised my hand, both hands, swooped them up and down like a golden gloves champion; stood up if necessary; jumped up if necessary, leaving papers and book flying; made all kinds of noises from intelligible, "Sister, *Sister*, SISTER!" to "Me, *Me*, ME!" to "I know, *I know*, I KNOW!" to unintelligible, "Eeennn, *Eeennn*, EEENNN; ssss, *Ssss*, SSSS; yahoww, *Yahoww*, YAHOWW!" Usually I was called on in these instances and performed beautifully. Occasionally, after all my gesticulations, I was called on and drew a blank. These blanks are my worst memories of school — exposed, nakedly stupid for all the world around me to see. Thank God, "my blanks" drove me to work harder, instead of quitting.

Even in explaining my three techniques, I have put the cart

before the horse. Often, very often, I couldn't decipher certain words when I tried to read them, or, deciphering them, I couldn't assign them meaning. How was it possible to work my way through this problem or, failing that, to fake my way through it?

At home, I developed a technique of playing word games until I got the information I needed. My family — especially my mother, God bless her — thought that I was playing fairly intelligent word games. Or else she knew I was faking and didn't admit it. My mother — God bless her again — had a way of caring without admitting or creating problems. Let me give you an example that I recall. I was reading an assignment when the words *reputable person* came along. *Table* I recognized; *repu* meant nothing.

"*Hey Mom, you know a lot about tables. Have you ever heard of a repoo-table?*"

"*No, Son.*"

"*I'm surprised because we had repoo-table in school today.*"

"*A repoo-table. You must be mistaken, Son.*"

"*How about a rep oo table?*"

"*No, Son, I guess you know something that I don't.*"

"*Is a person who owns a rep oo table a rep oo table person?*"

"*OK, Don. Another joke. You know that a reputable person is one whom people believe and trust.*"

"*I know that, Mom. I'm just joking with you.*"

With teachers, I had to play more subtle games. They didn't love me as much as Mom did. Here's an example.

"*Jane resides on Elm Street,*" I read.

"*What is Jane doing on Elm Street?*" I puzzled. "*Running? Climbing trees? Visiting? Selling lemonade?*"

No, the sentence would have said that. Let me check it out.

"*Sister, it says here that Jane re-sides on Elm Street. Why? Or why would Dick re-side on Oak Street or Mary re-side on Maple Street?*" (*Words that could be verified by concrete experience, like run, tree, lemonade, elm, were coming to me rather easily at this stage — but re-side?*)

"Stop trying to make things harder than they are. Why would anybody live where he lives?"

"Oh, sorry, Sister. Dumb question. Thank you."

And so I played, sometimes caught, more often not, as I got better at the game and more at home in this frightening, yet inviting, world of semantics. And so I worked and worked and worked. A lie here, an admission of guilt there, a triumph now and then, becoming more and more frequent. And so I climbed farther and farther away from my Eden of "just good ole me and good ole everything around me." My climb up the tree of word knowledge — grabbing abstract limb, finding footing on abstract branch, moving toward the fruit of contentment at the top — continued apace. But the fruit never got closer. It was only recently that I realized that the fruit was on the ground and I, for one, was letting it rot. The world of semantics has certainly been engrossing, but I have too often let it substitute for the enchantment of direct experience.

Something interesting and dismaying happened a few months ago. I got a phone call from Gary's mother. I had known Gary years before. He was an extremely bright and extremely learning-disabled young man. I showed him how to incorporate my techniques into his lifestyle and he conquered his learning disability. He graduated from high school and away he went into college, eager to climb the tree of knowledge and capture its fruit. That was the last I had heard from him or about him until his mother called.

"Gary," she said, "graduated from college a few years ago in a highly technical field. He got an excellent job."

"Great!" I said. I waited to hear about Gary's wife, maybe, and the beautiful kids.

"Gary," she continued, "was doing well on the job. He loved it. He had his own apartment. He was getting serious about a girl." Her use of the past tense alerted me to trouble, so I was ready.

"What happened?" I asked, expecting to hear about an accident.

"Now Gary has quit his job and has come back home. He won't leave his room. He's afraid to talk to anybody. He won't take phone calls. He won't eat with the family. He does occasionally get into long technical discourses about fields and particles that nobody can understand. I'm sorry to bother you, Mr. Lyman, but what have we here?"

"What have we here?" I thought. I felt I knew what they had there but I couldn't explain it to Mom. How could I say, "Ma'am, you have a semantic machine, perhaps a semantic monster in your house. He has let go of all that was real to him so completely, so finally (of course, he had to), that all he has left is words. Mom, you have become a word. Dad has become a word. Ambition, striving, success have become words. His girl friend has become a word. Technical operations have become words. He knows nothing anymore except words."

Instead, I said, "Let me talk to Gary." But Gary wouldn't come to the phone and I could understand that. How do you bandy words with some past apparition who told you words were important and who appears now, at Mom's behest, to tell you that words aren't so important, after all, and to get out there and confront reality?

I said to Mom all that I could say under the circumstances.

"Leave him alone for as long as he needs. Reality should return to him. If it doesn't after a while, get professional help."

When I write of Gary, I write of a minority so minuscule that it can hardly be expected to raise concern: a minority of dyslexics who have become living lexicons; learning disabled who can live only in a world of learning. There may be only one hundred or so of them in the whole country. People who look as if they're laughing when they cry because they forgot how to cry. People who look as if they're crying when they laugh because they forgot how to laugh. People who live vicarious, dictionary lives, expressing and defending themselves in words only because they have let go of real expression and real defenses long ago.

One thing has saved me. A thing called teaching. As teacher, I become vivacious, involved, stimulated, and stimulating — a real showman committed to the perfection of the performance and a super salesman committed to closure and results. Often I have heard, and still hear, other teachers comment on the change that comes over me when I enter a classroom.

Helping learning-disabled children overcome has indeed been the focus of my life. I have often weighed the consequences of not overcoming — the closed doors, the broken self-concepts, the withdrawal from effective participation in society, or the striking-back at a society that doesn't seem to understand or care. I comment on these things frequently in the ensuing pages. These consequences far outweigh the consequences of overcoming, for only a very few suffer from "word-sickness" and very many suffer the consequences of illiteracy. I mention the dangers of overcoming here only to make an obscure point clear. The learning-disabled child should not have to become a recluse, a fanatic for symbols, or an emotional mummy in order to overcome. This portion of my point is clear and easily accepted. The next part is not. The learning-disabled child should be accepted for what he is, admired for it, and encouraged to be himself.

First and foremost, he is a "real person" in a world chockfull of people, even full of children, who tend in varying degrees to be "unreal," to be aspiring or professional word manipulators. Second and secondarily, he is disabled, unable to function normally in a society that requires polished skill in reading, writing, speaking, and calculating. This disability must be overcome, but the chances of overcoming it are far greater when less effort is put into changing the child himself and more effort is made to enlarge his vision, showing him that from his concrete base and only from that base can he experience an enlarged world, albeit a semantic world. In my opinion, it is far better to feel exhilarated than to read about exhilaration, but it is better still to be able to experience it and also read about it. Vicarious exhilaration teaches new possibilities for happiness and sharing happiness. Yet without the base — with only the word — one does not really know what he is seeking for himself or seeking to share.

One day at recess, Jeff shouted to me.

"Come over here and see this. Hurry!" I went.

He was looking at a slender, striped lizard with a tail twice as long as its body.

"I've never seen a lizard like this before," Jeff whispered.

Now I knew quite a bit about lizards. I read about them because I knew that many of my students were interested in them.

"Sure you have. It's rather common. It's called a six-lined whiptail and . . ."

"Quiet."

Jeff was absorbed in watching the lizard scamper at phenomenal speeds for a short distance, tail swinging wildly, then come to a sudden halt, appearing dead, as if hit by a massive stroke. I was more interested in talking about it.

"It's also called a racerunner; it has . . ."

"Quiet."

"Notice how fine and smooth . . ."

"Quiet."

"Look at the stripes. Let's count . . ."

"QUIET!"

This was a rather loud and demanding "quiet," for the lizard had just come to life again, made a lightning move, and caught a very tiny frog in its mouth.

"That poor frog is a chorus frog. They . . ."

"Please, quiet!"

By this time, I was getting petulant. Who was this student to tell me, the teacher, to be quiet? I was already preparing the lecture I was going to give him about manners and understanding his place when I realized that he could have said "Shut *up!*" instead of "Quiet." I decided to let it go.

The lizard was now ingesting the frog. Only one leg remained outside its mouth.

"Both lizards and frogs have interesting digestive . . ."

"Shut up!"

That did it. "Jeff, I'm not going to take 'shut up' from you or anybody else. You've been looking for trouble and now you've found it."

"Jeez, Mr. Lyman. Did I say 'shut up'? I'm sorry."

"You're not going to get off with just an apology."

"OK. Punish me if it's so important to you. But remember, I asked you to come look at what was happening, not talk about it."

I remembered. He was right in what he said. He was also right in what he did. There is just no way to "capture a moment" in words, and Jeff had been trying to capture his moment with the lizard and frog. My words interfered.

"I'm ready for talk now," said Jeff. *"Tell me about the lizard and about the frog. I saw what happened. Now I want to know more."*

"OK, I'll tell you. But when I'm finished I'll think up some punishment. Students can't go around telling teachers to shut up under any circumstances."

"Hey, Mr. Lyman, how about making me write a compazishun [Jeff's usual spelling of the word] about lizards, all the different kinds."

"That sounds good. You can write a 150-word composition about lizards or a 25-word composition about manners. Take your choice."

"The lizards. The lizards. That ain't no punishment at all."

Jeff knew how to put "semantics" in its place, as well as me. Know something first in the concrete sense and then see what words can add to the experience.

Jeff was not an easy student. He came to my class at grade five and left three years later, moving to a different state. During those three years, he entertained and aggravated my other students constantly. Sometimes I felt as if he aged me six years during those three years. But three years after his departure, when he called to tell me how well he was doing in eleventh grade and how proud his parents were (confirmed by the parents), I wouldn't have cared, at the moment, if he had aged me six times six years. But I didn't express this special moment in words. If somebody had tried to speak to me just then, I probably would have said, "Shut *up!*"

So many Jeffs, Juans, Jeremys, Carolines, Larrys, and Franks over so many years. So much anguish. A little fat boy saying, "I'd rather be fat than stupid. Lucky me. I'm both." A tall, skinny, pimpled girl saying, "You know why I've got pimples? Because I'm not normal. Every time I can't figure something out another pimple breaks out. I'm so ugly but I deserve every goddam pimple on my face." Then mixed tears — half anger, half self-pity. An overactive, sweaty, clammy eight-year-old asking, "What's wrong with me? Every time I come in this classroom I feel like I can't breathe." A sixteen-year-old, veneered over with manners and appropriate behavior, suddenly throwing his book through a classroom window and then crying, crying, crying like a toddler who knocked over a pyramid of cans in a supermarket — afraid of the noise, afraid of the consequences. An adolescent girl, pretty face, so hunched over, almost deformed. Afraid to admit that she is pretty because as she says, "Retarded people aren't a pretty sight." Another girl, flaunting her body before every boy in class. "I may be stupid with books but this body you're seeing ain't no book; it's real. What you see is what you get."

And Jason, eleven years old, falling on the floor, faking seizures, faking death. Seeking attention and not caring what any adult or classmate thinks or says as long as he gets it.

Years of frustrating scenes, years of hearing "Books suck, but marijuana mellows," years of trying to help, often too little, too late. Brendan, a real, genuine person, high one night, driving his brain into his spinal column while showing off on a motorcycle; Leslie, runaway, found dismembered in a garbage can. And Gary, a success, home with Mom and Dad again, sitting in the same room he occupied as a child, shades drawn, doing absolutely nothing except thinking in words. Anguish, yes.

But there have been successes. College graduates, business executives, small business owners, commercial artists, teachers, foresters, auto mechanics, carpenters, contractors, engineers, hairdressers, pilots, blacksmiths, realtors, salespeople, interior decorators, karate experts, law enforcement officers, and on and on.

And there has always been the challenge. Help some and many more are waiting. Let go of the old group, some ready, some almost ready, some not ready at all. Take on the new group. Year after year the same. Year after year different, as real people, real children, find different ways of acting out their perennial question, "Why am I stupid when I know I'm not?"

I have lived with the problem of learning disability as far back as my memory goes. I have experienced it, I have taught thousands who have carried the label. Now I wish to share what I have learned.

Part Two

Reconsidering Special Learning Disability

4

What Is Learning Disability?

LEARNING DISABILITY has been with us as long as language, but only since 1962 (thanks to a special symposium at Johns Hopkins University) has it had the status of a specific handicap with specific symptomology, as well as a permanent label, Specific Learning Disability. Many other labels — some emphasizing particular aspects of the handicap, others trying to define the handicap by its cause (a difficult task, since its etiology is probably multiple and still unknown), still others trying to define it by eliminating the stigma of disability (also a difficult task because the handicap is very disabling) — have been used with varying degrees of acceptance. My latest count identifies fifty-five labels that have come along. Some have stayed; most have gone.

To identify the problem in this book, I will use Special Learning Disability, along with a standard definition:

> A disability occurring among people of normal intelligence, causing moderate to severe deficits in one, some, or all of the following: reading, spelling, writing, arithmetic, spoken language,* attention, concentration, memory, self-control, and/or organization.

*When oral-aural (expressive and receptive) language is severely limited this deficit area is sometimes given separate classification as Specific Language Disability.

Estimates of the number of children burdened by this handicap range from a conservative ten percent to an oversolicitous twenty-five percent. In any case, ten million to fifteen million of our children plus an uncountable number of adults experience learning disability. (Most adults tend to hide illiteracy, if possible.) These figures make Specific Learning Disability the most frequently occurring handicap in this country — most likely, in the world. And it is not a minimal handicap. It strikes at the very core of our humanness, depriving normal, creative individuals of their cultural birthright, stripping them of their sense of self-worth, diminishing or erasing their opportunities for satisfying participation in society. It is a handicap that drives many of our brightest children into a shadow world of drugs and crime.

A study conducted by the University of Colorado revealed that 80 percent of the prison inmates of that state had academic learning problems during their school years. Another study, made by the University of North Carolina, found that learning-disabled adolescents were three times more likely to choose a lifestyle involving illicit drug use, delinquency, and crime than other adolescents. The North Carolina study urged that the American judicial system make remediation of learning disability a top priority.

The medical, psychological, and educational communities, parent organizations, societies, and foundations have been addressing this problem with intensity for over two decades. I personally have addressed it, as a child and as a student, also as a parent of a learning-disabled child and as a teacher of other learning-disabled children. Specific Learning Disability has been interwoven into my life as far back as my memory extends. I invite you to accompany me as I revisit the learning-disabled child and reexperience and reexamine his handicap in the light of many small insights gained and discoveries and syntheses made during four and a half decades. Equally important, I invite you to become acquainted with the learning-disabled child on his own terms — on the basis of guarded and unguarded glimpses he has given me of his internal, subjective, very individual world.

I call the experience of this book a revisit, a reconsideration, not only because I review my own past experience but also because I approach that experience with fresh intuition and insight. Piaget points out that experience is not only receiving inputs but progressively constructing those inputs received. Each day, I learn from my continuing encounters with learning-disabled children.

Although there are advantages in having the label Specific Learning Disability, just a few weeks ago a twelve-year-old learning-disabled student announced to me that he didn't want to be called learning disabled anymore.

"I want that crossed out of my record," he insisted. "I have the right."

"What should be put in the record in its place?" I asked.

"Does anything have to be put there?"

"If nothing is there, they'll just put you back in a regular class. Maybe you'll fail reading, English, and math, as you did before. Then they'll think you're stupid and you know you're not."

"OK," he said, "put me down as temporarily learning something else."

This youngster was telling me two things about his disability: First, he assumed or at least hoped that someday he would master it. Second, in the meantime, he was not worthless or "put on ice." He was simply learning different things than most people learn (not necessarily in school) and in different ways.

5

Brain and Mind

THE BRAIN can be quantified. It can be divided into parts and parts within parts; divided into brain stem, medulla, pons, cerebellum, hypothalamus, thalamus, basal ganglia, limbic system, cortex, cerebral hemispheres, lobes, molecules, carbohydrates, fats, nucleic acid, DNA, RNA, ribosomes, amino acids, proteins. The mind cannot be quantified.

Philosophers, psychologists, theologians, neurologists, and biochemists have in their own ways tried to identify how mind relates to the brain or the cosmos or possibly both. Many theories — scientific, intuitive, metaphysical, and dogmatic — have suggested various relationships between mind and brain, but they are no more than theories. Behavioral psychologists in the last half century have told us that mind is really nothing. What we call mind, they call reflexes and conditioned responses. I don't believe that. I don't think some of them do either.

Very recently I had the opportunity to meet one of the most respected and published behaviorists in the country. He observed one of my classes and then told me (no connection between the observation and his words), "I really don't go all out for conditioning anymore. The area that must truly be examined is the cognitive, mental area."

Neurosurgeons, in spite of extensive brain mapping and probing, cannot tell us where mind exists. Psychologists cannot agree on its manner of functioning. The molecular structures that give rise to thinking, reasoning, concept formation, language, and emotion have their primary locus inside the skull, but mind is not the sum of these.

Mind is awareness of individual identity, motivation, strengths, weaknesses, goals, values, longings. It is self-concept, personhood. Mind is found through introspection and exercised through conscious choice. It can be glimpsed in a face straining to understand or to choose, or in eyes beaming delight or shielding deceit, in posture relaxed in confidence or slumped in despair. Only human beings can hate or love themselves; only human beings can pretend to be what they're not or pretend to have feelings that they do not feel. Only human beings have minds aware enough for this. Maybe only human beings have minds.

The brain thinks; the mind is aware that it is *I* who am thinking, about this, for this reason. The brain reasons; the mind is aware that it is *I* who am reasoning about that, for that reason. The brain structures language, but *I* speak and know what *I* am speaking about and *I* listen and know what *I* hear. The brain gives rise to feelings, but *I* feel them. The mind and the *I* are one.

It is my ability to maintain the integrity of my *I* that creates my personality. When my actions and my reactions, motives, goals, values, feelings, habits, language, skills, and relationships are fairly constant and predictable, I define myself to myself and to others. This personality as much as my physical appearance becomes associated with my name.

It is very difficult for the learning-disabled child to maintain the integrity of his *I*. Very often, his only predictable quality is his unpredictability. On certain days, he performs surprisingly well in class. His efforts produce immediate, short-term results. He is pleased with himself. His teacher is pleased. He tells Mom after school, "I had a good day." She is pleased. At home, he is less careless, less sloppy, remembers small responsibilities a little better. Things go smoothly. Mom is pleased. He tells his teacher the next morning, "I had a good night."

This does not happen very often. In spite of his best intentions, at school, his efforts to perceive symbols and understand semantics do not receive cooperation from his brain and body. At home, his nontemporal, illogical, nonsequential, "butterfly" lifestyle causes him trouble. Most of his days are bad days; most of his nights are bad nights. Most of those certain days that start good, turn bad. It is very easy for a good day to turn bad on him. It is almost impossible for a bad day to turn good.

The battle of mind-brain goes on constantly in and around the learning-disabled child. Consider these direct quotes from children I have taught. Not a word has been changed.

"My brain never does what I want it to do."

"I get something into my brain and my brain loses it."

"I don't know why I go to school. Nobody here can show me how to make my brain work right."

"I don't have a brain for this stuff" (reading comprehension exercise).

Most of these youngsters are very "down" on their brains. On their minds also.

As I mentioned earlier, it is difficult for the learning-disabled child to maintain the integrity of his *I*. Amid the conflict and pressure of his mind-brain warfare, he develops various styles of coping with internal and external realities. These styles manifest themselves as personalities, but he is not hypocritical; he is not schizophrenic. He is a person driven to maintain psychoneurological homeostasis and the scale keeps tipping.

Let me tell you about Frederick. I have his permission for this. He even suggested that I title the account, "The Three

Heads of Fred." In actuality, Fred has four heads or four *I*'s. First, there is struggling, volatile Fred. This is the Fred who tries to confront the reality of a school life chock-full of symbols and semantics and a home life characterized by very successful parents and siblings who demand like success of him. Struggling Fred approaches this reality with a furtive, haunted visage and a body locked into a fight-or-flight posture. When he makes the decision to try, it is a courageous decision, for he expects failure and further deterioration of his enfeebled self-concept. He can tolerate very little frustration; two or three small failures trigger his flight mechanism. (Fred always chooses flight over fight.) And Struggling Fred has become quite adept at flight. Place him at the starting line of the 100-meter dash in Olympic competition, ask him to read, and he will be a sure bet for a medal. He is shifty also. Place him in a starting backfield, ask him to spell a word in the huddle, give him the ball, and he'll run through and around a good defense that will look as immobile as eleven statues. When Fred chooses to run, desks, students, teachers, and bookcases are no obstacle. He is around them and out of the room with incomparable deftness. Struggling Fred lives a truly miserable, tapeloop life — decision, failure, flight — then courage to make another decision.

Second, there is Pretending Fred. This is the Fred who avoids confrontation; who sits quietly and pleasantly; smiles, pretends to listen, pretends to care, and does absolutely nothing. It is impossible to ruffle Pretending Fred. Admonitions, encouragements, threats, shouts, heart-rending pleas, promises of reward from the teacher, his fellow students, the principal, his parents called in for conference, even counseling psychologists do not reach him, much less penetrate him. Fred maintains a willful smile throughout and occasionally volunteers the brief paragraph that has become his hallmark.

"Don't get all worked up. I'm all right. I already know what you're trying to teach me. Take my word for it."

Eventually we turn behaviorist and seek to extinguish Fred's behavior by ignoring it. But he usually continues to pretend for days, even weeks. Then he decides to try again or he phases into *I* number three.

The third Fred is Concrete Fred. This Fred is delighted by anything — lizards, bugs, animals, fish, pencils, furniture, doors, windows, stairs, rails, vehicles, straws, microscopes, slides, pictures, drawings, puzzles, games, calculators, computers, things that stretch, things that break, scales, rulers, T-squares, test tubes, engines, machines, how the body works or breaks down, trees, bushes, flowers, weeds, how parts are put together, how wholes are taken apart, stopwatches, crustaceans, invertebrates, lakes, ponds, seas, weather, clouds, manual things, visual things, music, construction, destruction, beauty, ugliness, designs, angles, protractors, blackboards, chalk, Magic Markers, dirt, sand, stones, tools, sticks, yardsticks, containers, elements of electronics, projects, people (especially funny, happy, humming, unpredictable people) — anything except words. Concrete Fred becomes so immersed in the concrete world that one feels guilty drawing him away from it. Yet Concrete Fred will do his school assignments, not carefully, not often correctly, but willingly. He takes interest in the sweep of his pencil over the paper, in the quality of his erasures, in the overall appearance and design of his finished work. He will often augment this design with doodles, hexes, ornate letters that are fantastic and purposeless. Concrete Fred is affable, relaxed, and interesting. But his teachers and parents worry that he is not learning anything, that he is not being prepared for real life.

There is a fourth Fred, Introspective Fred. This is the one who monitors the other three; the one who decides which Fred will confront reality today.

Sometimes I talk with Fred. Not long talks. Fred is made uncomfortable by long talks. Once I asked him,

"Why do you ever try when you expect that you're going to 'mess up' every time?"

"I dunno. People expect it. Maybe I'll stop 'messing up.' "

"You don't have to be perfect, you know. When you make mistakes you don't have to run away."

"I know, but nobody makes as many mistakes as me. I can't stand it when I feel stupid."

"A lot of people make as many mistakes as you."

"Sure. Tell me again. So what? They don't mind feeling stupid."

"How should school be to make you happy?"

"I dunno. It's not my job to say how school should be."

"When are you happy?"

"I dunno. Sometimes. Sometimes when I do what I want."

"What are those things?"

"Anything that's not schoolwork. When I don't have to listen to words all the time, and spell and write and read words. They're boring for me. Can I go now?"

I let Fred go. Why pile more words on the fire? Imagine such a great distaste for words and a brain that won't process and remember them and a mind that forces itself to deal with them. Fred's mind-brain warfare on the battlefield of semantics is a warfare that every learning-disabled child wages — most to a lesser degree than Fred, some to a greater degree. But warfare in any degree is hell.

6

Perceiving and
the Mind-Brain

THE HUMAN MIND-BRAIN cannot perform its function of feeling, thinking, reasoning, concept forming, introspecting, and directing activity without connections to external reality, connections made by the senses (internal and external) and the efferent and afferent pathways of the central nervous system. Perception is not mind-brain activity alone; nor is it solely neurosensory activity. It is a composite of both. There cannot be a concept without a percept any more than there can be a heartbeat without blood. Neither does percept have any meaning without concept, just as blood lacks meaning without a heart to circulate it. Or using a different metaphor, it is difficult to imagine an "inscape" without a landscape or seascape. It is also difficult to assign much meaning to the beauty of landscape or seascape without at least one single mind to appreciate it.

Actually, perception is a series of composites. It is not only a composite of percept and concept but also a composite of present sensory impressions and memories of previous impressions. In the process of perception the present always meets the past. I cannot perceive the visual image of a bird without possessing the concept of "birdness"; nor can I perceive a bird at present in any meaningful way without immediately matching and mismatching my present bird with previous birds that I've perceived.

Perception is also a composite, a cross-indexing, of multiple sensory experiences. None of our senses stands alone. All of them are involved in the shaping of a perception. But perceiving is not only a matter of engaging different senses in sequence. Efficient perception demands that our senses operate simultaneously and instantly. I refer here not only to the external senses but also to proprioceptors, sense organs located in all the muscles and joints of the body. Proprioceptors send messages to the mind-brain just as the eyes and ears do. Telling the mind-brain of the body's position in space, relating body parts to each other as well as to external realities, proprioceptors must coordinate with each other and with the external senses if a perceived event is to be usable and understandable.

Everyone knows the story of Helen Keller. We can all recall her initiation into the world of words. The word *water* drawn on her hand by her teacher meant nothing to her until the teacher brought Helen to the water pump and splashed water over her hand. For Helen, sightless and soundless, this tactile and proprioceptive experience was enough. She was able to assign meaning to the word *water*. Helen was not "learning disabled."

Learning-disabled children see, hear, and feel, but words still do not make sense — especially words drawn on paper. Helen had only touch and proprioception to guide her. Not much coordinating or cross-indexing of senses was required, only an active mind. Learning-disabled children have active minds, but the cross-indexing of many sense impressions slows them down and even halts them. Feeling the water — as well as seeing it ripple and hearing it splash — is so primary, so fundamental, that reading and writing the word *water* suffers. Their central nervous system is geared to fundamental, not symbolic, experience.

In addition to previous composites, perception is also a composite of intake through sensory organs and outputs to them. When my eyes and mind-brain perceive a visual event (this is a simplification that omits a number of composites), the image of the event starts at the eye, is processed in the central nervous system, and must be fed back to the eye as a visual concept-percept so that its match with external reality can be verified.

Perception of language with its symbol system and related semantics introduces additional composites. In order to perceive aural language (language that I hear), I must coordinate a stream of phonemic percepts and simultaneously match these percepts (which are quite arbitrary) with previously perceived nonsemantic concepts. Paradoxically, this is the way I arrive at semantics.

Why should the word *bird* represent a very light, feathered creature that flies? Or why should the word *courage* represent the fearless yet fearful choices I make that make me a distinct person? Why doesn't *courage* fly or why don't I act *birdously*? It is all arbitrary, yet this is the nature of semantics. In order to think or reason, I must be able to coordinate and relate concepts (or words) with amazing facility. In order to speak I must accurately feed back these concepts to the proprioceptors of my vocal apparatus.

When I perceive visual language, I must match visual symbols with aural-oral phonemes, making a composite of a symbol with its symbol. To make matters more difficult, aural symbols do not consistently match with visual equivalents; in English there are more mismatches than matches. For example:

> boat should be bote
> boot should be bute
> team should be teme
> paid should be pade

right should be rite
route should be rute or rowt
judge should be juj
ledge should be lej
lodge should be loj

And you can think of hundreds of mismatches in addition to these. It is, of course, necessary that I simultaneously match my visual symbol of an aural symbol with a concept I already know in order to read words. If I wish to write, I must accurately feed back my perception to the proprioceptors of my arms and hands and to the external sense organs of my fingers. As you can see, perception is not a simple matter.

Ever since 1962, when the study brief from Johns Hopkins University bundled dyslexia (can't read), dysgraphia (can't write), and dyscalculia (can't do math) into a single syndrome, Specific Learning Disability, the word *perception* has been given extraordinary prominence. "Perception" had been an occasional visitor to various learning theories developed earlier in the century and in the previous century, but with the arrival of SLD, it not only came into its own but became ruler (sometimes tyrant) of numerous theories of "dyslearning." When a mother was previously told, "Ma'am, your son (or daughter) has a learning problem," it was something she could deal with. Make him study harder and longer, get a tutor, tan his little hide for being so lazy. But "Ma'am, your son has a perceptual problem (or a perceptual disorder or a visual-perception problem, or an auditory-perception problem, or a perceptual-motor problem, or a visual-motor-perception problem, or a perceptual-impulse disorder, or a sensory-perceptual disorder)" was more than she could deal with.

"Oh Lord, my son is handicapped. What will my husband think? (Fathers usually did not attend these early psycho-educational conferences. Now fathers and mothers are teaming up more often.) What will the neighbors think? Where do

I get help for a perceptual problem? Doctor? Psychologist? Physical therapist? Do I mortgage my house to pay for help? What did I do wrong? I remember he spoke late, didn't crawl, was very active, was a head banger, had awful tantrums. Why didn't somebody tell me sooner?"

Many new methods of teaching perception were instituted in the schools. Very few are still in use today. Perceptual-training centers proliferated from coast to coast. Very, very few of these are still in existence.

Cognitive approaches are more popular today. Concept is throwing out percept. This is not surprising since most perceptual training programs have been based on notions of perception that are too simplistic. And remember, perception is not a simple matter.

I do not feel that training in perception should be abandoned or even downgraded. My conviction is that concept and percept are one. In helping a learning-disabled child master his disability, it is wise, I feel, to start outside, move inside, and come back outside again to check on what happened inside. In this way, you bring together all the parts that must work as one in order to create a composite of what is sensed and what is meant.

In my work with learning-disabled children, I have dealt with the many composites of perception that I have described in this chapter. My own experiences and observation of the children themselves have confirmed that, while I may not have found the hiding place of the handicap, at least I'm "getting hot" in the hide-and-seek game of Specific Learning Disability.

Perception is a complex process and can break down at any one or more of these composites. It can also be constructed at these junctures. Let me give you some examples. *There, where, then, when, while, which, that, who,* and other similar words are notorious demons for learning-disabled children, who often misread or misspell these words well into their high school years and even into adulthood. *There* can become *ther* or *Thair* or *tere* or *thier*. *Who* can become *ho* or *hew* or, most often, *how*. I have seen all of these spellings. In addition, these words are often substituted for each other in reading or replaced by the simple *the*.

Is this a perceptual problem? Yes, partly. Most learning-disabled children have incomplete cerebral dominance (more about this in a later chapter). This causes an external "mixing up" of left and right and an unreliable reading from the internal compass (mind-brain proprioception) that monitors lateral direction and position in space. Many learning-disabled children have subtle balance problems that can affect the efficient perception of vertical direction. (Diagonal direction lies somewhere in between the two.)

Considering the directional confusion engendered by incomplete or "mixed" dominance, it is fair to say that some learning-disabled children are misperceiving the direction and sequence of the letters in words and that this misperception causes difficulty in word recognition and duplication. But there is more to it than this. Most learning-disabled children do not confuse direction when they draw concrete objects. Why the confusion when they write words? This brings us back to concepts and semantics. Letters are symbols used to construct concepts, to give oral and visual meaning to abstract notions. (A tree is not abstract; its concrete representation is the drawing of a tree. The word *tree* is abstract.) The learning-disabled child's inability to read and spell is caused by a breakdown of the concept-percept composite. With some children, perhaps the concept swallows the percept. "Tree" cannot be handled as an abstraction. Mind-brain converts it to a concrete multisensory image. The symbols go begging. With others, perhaps the percept swallows the concept. Mind-brain does not consider meaning at all, but becomes engaged in the spatial subtleties of the letters, even the empty spaces around them. Maybe some children are confused by both —

a double swallowing. Two perceptual snakes each swallowing the other's tail. A very confusing and uncomfortable situation. I'm sure that some learning-disabled children simply misperceive. And I'm sure some suffer from misperception as well as concept-percept indigestion. I must remind you again that perception is not a simple matter.

Let's return to the demon words I listed earlier. Why do these words cause special difficulty for many learning-disabled children? A girl named Michelle gave me the answer once. This eleven-year-old almost always misspelled and misread these words. When she didn't, it was the result of the purest luck, and she admitted it. Time-honored visual perception and sensory integration drills were no help to her. Copying the words five, ten, twenty, one hundred times did not help. She usually started misspelling them after the third time. One day I asked Michelle why she had so much trouble remembering these words.

"Because they don't have any damn meaning," she told me. What Michelle lacked in grace she compensated for in frankness. I decided to probe further.

"No meaning?"

"Yeah, when I begin to remember the dumb letters and put them together I can't picture them meaning anything. So I just forget the dumb letters."

(The concept swallowed the percept.) But what concept? Michelle said that these words had no meaning for her. This is the key. These words are symbols of empty categories. Categories that still have to be filled. They are temporal, spatial, relative, causal. Time for what? What's in the space? Relative to what? Causing what? Let me give some examples:

"*When* Joan arrived, she was horrified." In this form, the sentence means little to the learning-disabled child. If it were written, "Joan arrived and looked around. She was horrified" or "Joan arrived and heard the news. She was horrified," the child would have a much better chance at reading it meaningfully.

or

"The book is *where* you left it" would make more sense to the learning-disabled child as, "Did you leave the book on a desk, in the closet, or under the bed? Go look."

or

"The person *who* practices the hardest should win the prize." The word *who* is an empty category for the learning-disabled. It would be easier for them to read and comprehend if it were restated as, "Practice hard and you can win. Let anybody practice hard and he can win. Practicing hard is very important" — or something similar.

or

"*Since* John was sick, he didn't go to school today" should be rephrased for the learning-disabled as, "You don't see John in school today. He's sick."

So much of our language, of any symbolic language, is hung together and strung together by words that are empty categories waiting to be filled — words that make little sense alone, but, when placed in sentences, create essential relationships. But the very concrete learning-disabled child cannot wait. Neither does he find it easy to move ahead and then look back to see the relationship. By that time, the word has become empty again. Concreteness is a "now" kind of thing and must be satisfied here and now.

I said earlier that perception is a composite of present sensations and memory of past sensations. Let me illustrate this. Once, very early in a long-gone school term, eight-year-old George made the following request: *"Sir, please move me up to the next book. This one is too easy for me."* What George lacked in frankness he made up for in grace. I knew that he could barely read the book he had.

"George, read me some of that book and I'll decide if you know it well enough to move up."

"Sir, it will be a waste of time. I already know it."

"I don't doubt that you know it, George. (I did doubt it and George knew that I did.) Just read me a little so I can be sure before I move you up."

"Isn't it time for recess, sir?"

"Almost, but we still have time. Here, I'll just open to any page and you start reading."

"I have a little headache, sir."

"Reading will help it to go away."

"Sir, I'm just not in a reading mood today."

The recess bell rang. George won that skirmish, but I eventually won the war. The very next day I convinced George to read. The feat wasn't easily accomplished. I won by attrition. George pulled every trick from his bag of excuses. His best was:

"Sir, my mom told me not read for a few days because of a blister in my mouth."

"Let me see the blister."

"I'm not supposed to get air on it."

"Let's call your mother and get permission."

When George exhausted his bag, he had nothing left except stubborn refusal without any excuses, running from the room (like the first head of Fred), or reading. He had too much decorum to choose either of the first two alternatives. Besides, he was chunky and not very fast. I would have caught him easily. He chose to read.

It was a pitiful attempt. He did not get past the fifth word (all of which I supplied) when he broke down completely. I have never seen tears burst out so relentlessly. They did not come singly but in puddles. Within seconds his entire face and both hands were wet. He cried:

"Sir, they never taught me to read in first grade and every time I try, I think of first grade. I keep getting worse, not better."

George was saying in his way that he did not learn to perceive visual-aural symbols accurately during his first year in school and that his present attempts were only building additional confusion on top of a confused past. Every time he tried to learn to read, he was adding another layer of confusion to his perceptual apparatus. Certainly something to cry about. Especially at age eight.

By the way, George did become a reader before the year was over. During the next year he achieved proficiency.

I mentioned earlier that perception is a composite of multiple sensory experiences. The different sensory avenues must coordinate in the mind-brain in order to perceive accurately and efficiently. Like workers on an assembly line, they must complement each other. If they don't they will set each other off like siblings doing the dishes.

Consider ten-year-old Whitney, who is trying to read in my class. He sees a word. It must be hard for him because he keeps seeing it but doesn't say it. He blinks away from the word. My guess is that he is trying to visualize the word (see it in his mind). He brings his finger to the word and glides the finger back and forth beneath it. Now his eyes become steadier and I see his lips moving, but he still isn't saying anything. My guess is that he is auditorializing. He is trying to think the sounds of the word in his mind as he zeros them in with his finger and is calling on the muscles and nerves of his vocal apparatus to help. As his lips slow down, he begins to stare at the word again and move his shoulders from side to side. His head bends down close to the word, his finger becomes quite active, sometimes stabbing at the word, and his lips pick up their pace again. Even his feet begin to tap. My guess is that visualizing, auditorializing, plus a little bit of neuromuscular support failed him, so he is in the process of calling up additional reinforcements from his neuromuscular arsenal (proprioception). He even bends so close to the book that I almost expect him to bite it. None of this helps. He looks up in despair and I give him the word. Eyes focus, lips stop moving, body settles down, and he reads the word as if he knew it all of his life. But then begins the encounter with new words.

When I give Charlie, age ten (a lend-lease from a regular

class), the same reading assignment, he reads the word and many more without blinking, moving lips, jerking hands, or tapping feet. Why? Is Charlie more intelligent than Whitney? Hardly. Whitney's current IQ is 119. Charlie's is 97.

This phenomenon, I'm sure, cannot be explained in terms of sensory incoordination alone. But judging from Whitney's behavior it would be a disservice to the learning-disabled child to discount it. You see, most of the learning disabled I have taught have approached the reading task just as Whitney did. Many of the minority who did not simply sat and stared at the reading text. In my opinion, these children overcontrolled the "Whitney-type" reading behavior, moving themselves one step further from eventual mastery of the skills necessary for reading.

Sensory coordination means more than using a multisensory approach. Whitney engaged every sense available to him short of trying to smell meaning from the word; yet these did not help him. A principal reason that Whitney failed in his reading task was that he had not learned the skill of using his senses all together as a composite, in a gestalt operation, as a part of the unified process of perception. And if senses do not unite in simultaneous effort, they interfere, distract, impede, and confuse. How often as a teacher, I have seen a youngster try to concentrate on what I was writing, while my words and his very own body position and movements were distracting him from learning. How often I have seen a youngster try to concentrate on what I was saying, while the very things I wrote to reinforce my words (as well as the movement of my arm while writing them) distracted him from learning.

Whitney did eventually learn to coordinate his senses in the act of perceiving symbolic language, and his reading showed its greatest improvement after the acquisition of this skill.

One final aspect of my perceptual construct that I would like to discuss in this chapter I call perceptual feedback.

When a learning-disabled child reads orally, he must "take in" visual symbols, match them with auditory equivalents that are already in the mind-brain, add on a layer of meaning, and feed all of this back to his vocal apparatus as well as to his eyes. In this way he can be sure that he is saying the word he sees. Unfortunately, he often says the wrong word or no word at all. When a learning-disabled child takes a spelling test, he must take in auditory symbols, match them with visual equivalents that are already in the mind-brain, add on a layer of meaning, and feed all of this back to the proprioceptors and tactile organs of hand and finger in order to write. Likewise, he must send feedback to the vocal organs to reinforce the act of writing. In this way he can be sure that he is writing the word that he heard. Unfortunately, he often spells the word incorrectly or writes nothing at all. Such breakdowns in completing the perception cycle can occur at many points. The point of feedback is only one, but it is worth considering. Let me illustrate.

On occasion I conduct spelling bees for learning-disabled children. I do my best to organize the bees into successful learning experiences. The children practice the required words with great determination in preparation for the bee. During the bee, the student may either say the word or write it on the board. He is given five chances to self-correct, with hints being given at each correction. If he still misses after five tries, I write the word on the board, let him glance at it briefly. Then I erase it and he tries again. You can see why these spelling bees usually last all morning. Many of the excuses I hear from the children as they make mistakes relate to feedback:

"*I had the word in my head and lost it.*"

"*I knew it. I know I knew it. It was right on the tip of my tongue.*"

"*Why did I write that dumb word? That's not what I meant to write.*"

"If you could just see inside my head, you'd know that I know it."

"These [bleep] words never come out right."

There is no question that short-term memory is a factor here. But these children do not appear to be blaming their mistakes on memory alone. They are also blaming an inability to "get it out." If we can rely on the message these youngsters are giving, remediative procedures with learning-disabled children should include procedures and practices that address the feedback mechanisms of perception.

I have said repeatedly in this chapter that perception is a complex process composed of many composites and that it can break down for learning-disabled children at any single composite or combination of them. It is important to add that perception can also be constructed or learned at each of these junctures. Part Four of this book suggests ways that this can be accomplished.

7

Seeing and the Mind-Brain

THE EYE AND MIND-BRAIN COMBINATION is fascinating because it presents some fascinating questions, especially to the teacher or parent of a learning-disabled child. Why, for example, is your dog, Thor, brought by your eye's lens to the retina as an upside-down, mirrored image, yet Thor is seen in your mind right side up? Why is he seen in actual size when his image on your retina is tiny? And why do you see him out there, leaving fleas on your carpet, when the image is in your mind? Why does the SLD child focus on the letter *d*, receive it on his retina as *9*, yet see it in his mind and on the page sometimes as *d*, sometimes as *b*, sometimes as *g*, sometimes as *p*, maybe even as ⌐◖ or ▬◖? Why does his mind see the *d* in sizes that can vary from the actual print? I have heard different learning-disabled children insist that *d* , *d* , and *d* are all the same size, especially when they were the ones who wrote the *d*'s.

Over twenty-five years ago, an experiment was designed at the University of Wichita (now Wichita State University) to seek answers to some of these questions. The experimental subject was fitted with lenses that not only inverted the image but reversed it. In the case of this poor subject, not only did up become down, but right became left. He wore the lenses during all waking hours and slept with patches on his eyes at night — for one complete month. During this time he was asked to do small muscle tasks like walking floor mazes. In addition to this, he had to handle normal tasks such as walking around and eating. He even drove a car. One of the conclusions drawn from the subject's performance of the experimental tasks was:

> During the thirty-day period that the inverted lenses were worn, the visual-motor coordinations were refashioned in the central nervous system so that the subject performed even better than before the lenses were put on.

Let me put it another way. During the thirty-day period the subject's mind-brain made a complete adjustment that enabled him to perceive things as he had perceived them since infancy — out there and right side up with the left wall to his left and the right wall to his right. If he turned, he had to reorient his internal compass, for what used to be the left wall might now be the wall in front of him. When he was an infant he had no words for this, but his eyes, body, and mind-brain knew. Infant eyes wander, then look at something. Touch it. Hands wander, then touch something. Look at it. Learn to look at and touch at the same time. Turn, and it is easier to use the other hand. Maybe the other eye. Yes, the infant learns he has two of them. A little older and fall — bump! Again and again. Now he knows down and he can reach up to get up. Much learning takes place without a single word.

This quaint old experiment was not performed with learning disability in mind, nor is it mentioned in any learning-disability research to my knowledge. Yet I feel that it has important lessons to teach us.

Lesson One: Until about twenty years ago, it was assumed

that a youngster who reversed, omitted, substituted, inverted, mirrored, or otherwise misread or miswrote letters was
suffering from a vision problem. And why not? It seemed obvious that he was seeing the letters incorrectly. His condition
was called word blindness or symbol amblyopia. Various
forms of ocular motor training became the favored therapy,
mainly because something had to be done and nobody was
sure what else to do. Today, most will agree that ocular motor
training alone is without merit for reading or writing dis-
orders.

About the time that ocular therapy was most prominent, I
was doing a little informal in-class experimenting. I was
teaching various groups at that time and concentrated my
experiment on a six- to eight-year-old group, most of whose
members were only beginning to remember letters well
enough to read and write. After writing a letter on the board,
I would ask my students to take a good look at it, then close
their eyes, and see it inside their heads. Now, learning-disabled children don't lie any more than other children and
often less in stressful situations. What I usually got in response was, "I can't, I can't" coming from frustrated children
all over the room. The occasional "I can see it" came either
from the exception or from youngsters like George who felt
compelled to cover up their disability at almost any cost.

I verified their difficulty to my own satisfaction by writing
a letter or two on the board, asking the students to study carefully what I had written and warning them that I would soon
erase the letter and expect them to remember "how it went."
I let the students tell me when they felt they were ready. Then
I erased and asked them to write the letter or letters. They
couldn't write a single letter accurately most of the time. It
was extremely rare that they could write two. My own experience in the elementary grades was further verification. I recalled trying to learn the spelling of very simple words by
picturing their individual letters in sequence in my mind. The

only way I could force my stubborn brain to cooperate was by actually "punching out" the direction of each stroke made in writing the letter. For example, if I were trying to visualize the manuscript* letter Ⓠ , I would punch with my left fist to the left; next I would punch downward with my left fist; then I would punch right with my right fist; finally I would punch up and down with my right fist — all of this with my eyes closed. The pattern I followed for this letter was:

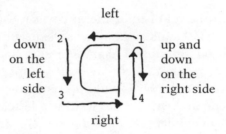

To begin with, all I could remember was this pattern, but I was delighted that I could see the lines of the Ⓠ forming inside my head as I did it. With much effort and much time, I eventually developed patterns for all twenty-six letters. Other learning at home and school was going on during this time, but my discovery was my "ace in the hole." When I couldn't remember a word in any other way, I punched it out until I could. I developed patterns for all letters. With each punch the corresponding line would appear "inside my head." The harder I punched the clearer the line appeared. After sufficient "punching out" of each letter of a word, I found that I could visualize the entire word without punching. I never "punched out" words in class. Being called Punchy by my peers would have destroyed me as much as being tagged Stu-

---

Manuscript writing is writing that consists of unjoined letters made with lines and circles and that is often taught in elementary schools.

pid. But I did a lot of private punching at home. It's a wonder
I didn't choose boxing as a career instead of teaching.

All of the above made clear to me that most learning-disabled children could not visualize symbols. I decided to try
making the symbols concrete. We chose a few letters, *A, t, c,
g, p.* I asked the children to find ways to make the letters into
real things. We finally settled on:

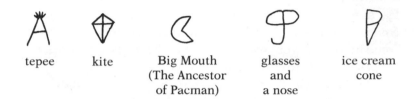

| tepee | kite | Big Mouth (The Ancestor of Pacman) | glasses and a nose | ice cream cone |

We stopped calling the letters by their symbolic names; we
used only the concrete names. In a very short time, all of the
children could duplicate all of the above objects not only individually but as a set. Many of the duplications were very
accurate. All were recognizable. My conclusion: Most learning-disabled children cannot visualize symbols; they can visualize concrete objects. This makes sense. These children are
very "concrete" creatures. Yet I could not very well use *tepee*
or *kite* or *big mouth* for semantic classroom instruction unless
I was ready to convince the world to accept into its culture a
separate picture language for the learning disabled. No
chance. Humanity was already convinced that symbolic, semantic language was what raised it above the caveman and
his near look-alike, the ape. No regression allowed here.

I knew, however, that I must teach these children to visualize symbols. I was convinced that the ability to visualize
was the key to visual memory and that I would not be able to
teach my class to read and write without this key. So I turned
to "punching out" letters as an aid to visualizing them. This
procedure proved so successful that I use it to this day. (It has

undergone many refinements. I will describe the current procedure in Part Four of this book.) I have theorized about the success of this procedure many times. Learning-disabled children *must* learn symbolic/semantic language. How do you help a child who has little difficulty visualizing and understanding concrete reality make the quantum jump to visualizing and understanding a string of symbols? It took millennia for mankind in general to make the jump. The learning-disabled child has only a few years at most to become acculturated in a literate society, and he will often become an awful problem to himself and society if he does not.

Let's concede that this child can visualize concrete objects. How do we make a symbol concrete for him without destroying the very nature of the symbol? It can't be done. No kind of logic has been found that can resolve absolute contradictions. (Except, perhaps, quantum logic, but most of us aren't ready for that jump.) If there is an answer, I theorized, it must be the product of some illogical thought process. Let's think together illogically.

Visualization must be a function of vision (the sender) and mind-brain (the receiver). Very logical. Learning-disabled children apparently visualize concrete objects according to this logic because they do this quickly and efficiently. These same children (unable to visualize abstract symbols) can make these symbols subjectively concrete by adding muscle and joint activity to vision and mind-brain. Clearly illogical. Yet the sense organs (proprioceptors) of the muscles and joints would appear to reinforce, even align, the efforts of eye and mind-brain in the process of perceiving letters. If these children can sense — can actually feel in their muscles and joints — the strokes needed to visually represent a letter, their central nervous systems allow them to image that letter and often to retain the image, just as they retain concrete images. Totally illogical. But effective.

Let's backtrack to the University of Wichita experiment.

The subject of the experiment spoke of his *visual-motor* coordinations being refashioned *in the central nervous system*. This statement implies that the subject's mind-brain made up become up again and down become down; that it made right become right again and left become left. Then it forced this information on the eyes confused by the inverting and reversing effect of the lenses. It also implies that a motoric (muscle, tendon, joint) input was involved, for the coordinations were visual-motor. The subject's mind-brain might not have made the complete adjustment that enabled him to see things as they were positioned in objective reality *if he had not moved around.*

Thus, Lesson One taught by the Wichita experiment — as far as learning disability is concerned — is that the visual symbolic misperceptions of learning-disabled children can be corrected by teaching them to visualize. Simply stated, when a learning-disabled child learns to picture individual letters and words in his mind, he will eventually stop reversing them, substituting them one for another, or omitting them. No more *bad* for *dad, wow* for *mom, horse* for *house,* or *sumr* for *summer.* Keep in mind that I am speaking only of perception here. Cognition (understanding words and their structure) will be dealt with later. The ability to visualize symbols can be assured by movement exercises that coordinate with the sequences of direction used in duplicating symbols.

Hold on for one final thought on this. You may think that writing is movement that coordinates with the sequence of direction in duplicating symbols. Won't writing teach the ability to visualize and retain symbols? Won't copying letters and words over and over do the trick? My answer is yes, eventually. But not at the beginning. Remember that I had to "punch out" direction in order to visualize and retain symbols well enough and long enough to learn how to read, spell, and write. And the harder I punched the clearer the vision. Well, writing just isn't "punchy" enough for us learning disabled. It is too fine and too weak to cause "imprinting" — at least at first.

Lesson Two: One aspect of the Wichita experiment stands out in my mind. This was an *intense* experiment. The subject did not wear the inversion lenses for forty-five minutes a day or for an hour three times a week. I doubt that his mind-brain ever would have made the adjustment to objective reality under those conditions. He wore the lenses continuously, every waking moment for one month.

I doubt also that the mind-brain of the learning-disabled child can make the adaptations necessary to perceive symbols accurately and overlay them with meaning unless he works at it *intensely*. In my opinion, some intervention here, some there, a little bit now, more later (even using very effective procedures), is as much a disservice to the learning-disabled child as the use of ineffective procedures. If the learning-disabled child is to master his handicap, it must be a full-time, all-day job (school and home in cooperation). Isn't intensive, hard work over the short run preferable to the chronic pain of handicap?

I have misgivings about part-time programs for learning-disabled children. Today, part-time help in teaching is called resource programming. The child spends part of his day receiving special help and part coping and compensating in regular classes. The part spent in regular classes is called mainstreaming. If the choice were mine, I would place these children in self-contained units, encourage development of their strengths, remediate their deficits, using the most effective procedures in a most concerted manner. Then after six months, a year, longer for some, I would transfer these children to the mainstream with an ability to compete, to run the race. I fear that resource-mainstreaming, part-time programs may teach these children an attitude of coping with literate culture, an attitude of adjustment to their handicap. I feel certain that learning-disabled children, made aware of the choice, would pick mastery over adjustment every time. Those I have worked with have chosen mastery. Many, many have achieved it. I chose mastery too.

Lesson Two teaches that perceptual deficiencies relating to Specific Learning Disability can be overcome only by long-term, day-in/day-out training directed at these deficiencies. Many hours a day for a month is far superior to three hours a week for a year. I have suggested a way to do this training in this chapter. In Part Four, I will explain the method in greater detail.

8

Hearing and the Mind-Brain

ON FIRST TAKING THOUGHT, we would not expect the mind-brain-ear function to be similar to the mind-brain-eye function. Further thought, however, reveals how amazingly the functions of these two combinations parallel each other. Sound and sight are so totally distinct, such different dimensions of sensation, that one would expect the mind-brain to handle them in different ways. It is true that they relate in the real world. Some sights emit sounds, or, for auditory types, sounds tracked down will emit sights. But this fact does not make the emissions any more similar. Our attention to the dissimilarity of the two sensations shows itself in the terms we use in dealing with learning disability. We speak of visual *perception*, but of auditory *discrimination*, as if the mind-brain has a different pattern in dealing with vision than it does with hearing. Actually, my experience shows me that mind-brain plays the same kinds of tricks on unfortunate learning-disabled children when it receives sensation from either sensory channel. Children commit the same kinds of reversals, omissions, substitutions, and additions in their aural/oral language as they do in their visual/written language. It is true that aural misperceptions often occur in conjunction with visual ones and that solely visual misperceptions are more frequent than purely aural. But aural misperceptions, pure and pristine, do occur with significant frequency. Since their patterns are so similar to visual patterns, I will use the term *auditory perception* rather than *auditory discrimination* to make clear that in dealing with both we are dealing with the same kind of mind-brain phenomenon.

Here is some evidence for my assertion: I use a procedure in teaching phonemes (sound clusters) to learning-disabled children in which I pair each of the short vowel sounds with each consonant (I do the same with long vowels and variants) and ask the students to tell me a word that has that sound in it. This is an auditory exercise. I coordinate it with reading and writing at a later stage. For example, I will say "ac." Some students will answer "act" or "acrobat"; a few will answer "cab" (pure auditory reversing).

I say, "Give me a word that has ab *in it; a few answer 'bad.' "*
"Give me a word with ub; *some answer 'but.' "*
"Give me a word with it; *a few answer 'tip.' "*

All are auditory reversals, as glaring as any reading or writing reversal. The reversal culprits are not always the same small group of children. I can expect a reversal sound from anywhere in the room; from a youngster who had been performing perfectly as well as from one who had been having difficulty. Most learning-disabled children reverse sound symbols at one time or another, just as they reverse visual symbols.

I have often listened to learning-disabled children speak words with omitted sounds.

"Rember *what happened yesterday."*
"Dad's angry because the *spinkler* system broke."
"I'll shove it down your *trowt (or* throw*)."*
"I didn't do *noten."*

The final *d* sound is a favorite for omission:

"This morning when I *answer* the phone . . ."

"After she open the door . . ."

Many of these children occasionally substitute sounds when they speak:

"All time ago . . ."

"Put it on the dable."

"That planned has a pretty flower."

They add sounds, too:

"How many exhamples do I have to do?"

"We bought a new lawnsmower (or sailsboat)."

"It's stuck up on the rooft."

You may think that all of the above are examples of articulation problems, caused by carelessness, anatomy, emotion, or local pronunciation. There are plenty of articulation problems, both among the learning disabled and learning abled that should be treated by speech therapists or language pathologists. But this is not what I am describing here. Neither am I describing a difficulty in applying grammatical rules. I am saying that many learning-disabled children have the same kind of difficulty internalizing symbolic/semantic sound (hearing it inside the head, auditorializing it) as they have in visualizing printed symbols; that the mind-brain of the learning-disabled child handles (or mishandles) both kinds of input in the same way. I am also convinced that auditory-perception and visual-perception problems can be treated similarly and should be treated in coordination.

Undoubtedly, some learning-disabled children can use their eyes better than their ears. Some are stronger auditorially. Observation of this fact has created the popular terms *visual* and *auditory* learner. It is my opinion, however, that learning disability cannot be mastered as long as either component remains weak. True, we should build on strengths, but we should also strengthen weaknesses. This is best done by coordinated effort, where the strong paves the way for the weak.

Let's discuss treatment.

In the previous chapter, I stated that an ability to visualize effectively was tantamount to perceiving effectively. I also mentioned that most learning-disabled children can visualize concrete objects but many cannot visualize abstract symbols. I then described how a muscle input or proprioceptive tie-in can, in a sense, make these symbols concrete so that they can be visualized.

In my judgment, all of the above points apply to auditory as well as visual perception. For years, parents of children with perceptual problems were given three pieces of advice:

1. Check the child's visual and/or hearing acuity (good advice).
2. Check for organ defects or deficits (good advice).
3. If the first two don't check out (in most cases there is no physical problem), get the child into a visual- or auditory-training program (dubious advice, if you expect perceptual mastery from the single intervention).

The third recommendation was especially dubious when auditory training was prescribed, not because the idea or intention wasn't good, but because nobody (even the therapist) was too sure what auditory training was. About fifteen years ago, I was teaching two students who happened to be enrolled in the same auditory-training program. When I saw no improvement in auditory perception after a number of sessions I decided to go to a session to observe. The children were given a worksheet with pictures of a train, a bell, a bird, a car, a cow, a dog, a bike, a whistle, and other things I don't remember. They were instructed to put on earphones and write a check next to the appropriate picture every time they heard a "tweet tweet," a "moo," a "woof woof," a "varoom," or whatever. I asked if I could participate too and was given permission. We all had a great time anticipating the sound that was coming. The children were correct with every check, even when the recording was speeded up. I missed a couple because I was worried about being a teacher who wasn't supposed to make mistakes and because I became distracted by watching the children enjoy themselves so much.

Then the task changed. We were instructed to check "same" or "different" as the machine vocalized pairs of vowel and consonant sounds in different combinations. The children were no longer having fun, for they were incorrect almost as many times as they were correct. When the recording speeded up, I knew that they were guessing most of the time. Chance ruled rather than perception.

The concept underpinning this procedure was that in learning to discriminate concrete, nonsymbolic differences in sound, the child would develop an ability to discriminate subtle symbolic differences. That just because he could tell a train whistle from a dog's bark, he could tell "dog" from "dug" or "pet" from "pit." Not so. These children could already discriminate the concrete sounds. Learning disability involves misperception of *symbolic* language, not concrete language. Hearing Sally sigh is not the same as hearing the words, "Sally's sighs made me sympathize with her all the more." The learning-disabled child might be thinking of legs. The procedure was also built on another misconception, a misconception that still influences many practices in use today. The misconception: visual perception can be taught by practice in visual perception; auditory perception can be taught by practice in auditory perception. You do *not* correct misperception by practice in selecting correct perceptions from a series of incorrect ones or incorrect perceptions from a series of correct ones. "Practice makes perfect" does not apply here. "Practice creates confusion" does. A child who does not "see" or "hear" symbols correctly, does not because he cannot. Showing him or telling him what is correct in contrast to what he incorrectly perceived does *not* correct the problem. He may be "misperceiving" the correct symbol as you applaud its correctness. A common practice in learning-disabled circles is to ask the child to choose one word that matches the end sound of a lead word. He must read the words but concentrate on matching the sounds. For example:

> Set: sit, put, met, bat, lot
> Lonely: only, fondly, bone, silly, lovely

This kind of exercise is mind-brain poison to the learning-disabled child — a fatal eye-blurring, ear-scrambling mixture of similar sights and sounds with no hint given about the meaning of any of them. He may choose *met* because he compares the *ets* visually, having no idea how they sound; or he may choose this word because, if you flip *s* on its belly, it looks a little like *m*; or because *met* is in the middle. He may choose *only* because he's too tired to look beyond the first word; or because *lonely*, without the *l*, looks like *only*; or because it is the shortest word except for *bone*, but *bone* doesn't end in *y*; or because he remembers "Only the Lonely" from a record album. His "process for perceiving" does not function for him. This is what must be corrected.

I know that the learning-disabled child can perceive differences in pitch, intensity, tone, and timbre among sounds that have a concrete source and purpose. I have used tapes with many of these sounds and my students have easily identified them. I also know that many of these children have difficulty perceiving (discriminating and using) symbol-related sounds. I have taped sounds of the outdoors. Birds chanting, different birds in different keys and pitches — sweet, raucous, and plaintive. Construction site noises — hammering, drilling, metal on rock. Nature's sounds — thunder, hard rain, soft rain, surf, wind passing through trees. On the same tape, I recorded the sound of "ĕ," as in *pet*; "ă," as in *pat*; "ŭ," as in *put*; "ŏ," as in *pot*; "ĭ," as in *pit*; "th," as in *through*; "br," as in *bring*, "ow," as in *how*; "ain," as in *rain*. I have played these tapes to classes. Almost without exception, the children have

been able to identify every concrete sound. With few exceptions, they could not handle symbolic sounds.

"Sounds like a fart."

"Sounds like a burp."

"Sounds like something real sick made that sound."

"Sounds like nothing."

*"Sounds like those stupid sounds they use when they teach
phonics."*

Some joking in these answers. Some attempt to show me
what they thought of symbolism. But no discrimination. If
they could have discriminated the sounds, they would have
let me know for sure.

"That's an 'aah' like in 'saaht' (sat).

"That's an 'eeh' like in 'seeht' (set).

For learning-disabled children, a small success rates higher
than a big joke. But there were few small successes to be
found in this instance.

Can these children auditorialize concrete sounds (hear
them internally)? Yes. They hear the sounds and can duplicate them. Maybe, you can argue, they are simply parroting
or echoing the sounds. What proof is there that they are actually hearing these sounds inside? My proof lies in the fact
that the children can repeat the sounds after a few moments
or minutes. They certainly do not hold the sounds "in their
heads" during this period of time. They must be able to res-
urrect and hear them with the mind's ear before repeating
them.

But not only do these children have difficulty auditorializing symbolic sound. They are not consistent in their ability to
repeat these sounds after hearing them. They are even less
consistent in their ability to remember and retrieve them.

I am convinced that ability to auditorialize opens the door
to accurate auditory perception. But how does one teach this
ability?

The first clue comes from my private practice sessions during my own elementary school years. In order to reinforce my ability to "think" letter sounds (especially short vowel sounds, which were the ones that caused me most difficulty), I used five words that had become almost concrete to me. These words became objective referents during my self-created (and self-inflicted) auditory-training sessions. I used the word *sin* for the short "i" sound. This word had been practically imprinted in my nervous system by the zealous, God-fearing nuns. For short "u," I used the word *tub*. I was really into baths. They were a sure way to gain privacy during my more silly training workouts. In the tub I could also practice oral reading without fear of failure. Besides, I like water, especially hot water in winter. For the short "a" sound I used *mad*. I was good at thinking this word since somebody always seemed to be mad at me. Especially for staying in the bathroom too long. For short "o" I used the word *fog*. This word had achieved concrete significance for me a couple of years earlier during a family auto trip. My father was driving through a dense predawn fog so thick that I could see nothing outside the car. I wondered how he could drive at all. I felt extremely lonesome even in the company of my sleeping family. I was fearful, confused, blinded to everything around me. I felt lost in a gray obscure sea; the feeling perfectly matched a similar feeling that sometimes overwhelmed me in the classroom. Suddenly I would feel fearful, confused, blinded, lonesome; alone on a raft in the bookish (semantic) sea surrounding me. The sound *fog* was easy to remember.

For the short "e" sound (the sound most difficult for me), I used *Fred*, the name of my best friend. Fred was a loner, a weird sort of person, forever finding or inventing gadgets that were a lot of fun to play with. I was very fond of Fred. I could never have called him Frid, Frad, Frod, or Frud. The sound *Fred* was easy to remember. Starting with these definite words that contained definite sounds, I would match their vowel sounds in my head with various consonants in a chain of nonsense combinations. For example, I would think "sin," then follow this thought with "ininipibicidisim" as quickly as the consonants would occur to me.

tub — ŭbŭbŭpŭnŭmŭsŭt
fog — ŏgŏgŏtŏjŏnŏlŏbŏcŏv
mad — ădădăbătăcăfăp
Fred — ĕdĕdĕpĕtĕgĕnĕmĕl

And so I would go. Often I sang the nonsense sounds in my mind. Then I sang them out loud for external confirmation. Singing was much more fun than simply saying. After some time at this, I would search for words in reading assignments that had the same sound combinations and read them with great satisfaction. Sometimes I read them correctly, sometimes incorrectly. Variant sounds for these letters got the best of me. It was some time before I began to master them.

The above procedure was helpful but became more worthwhile and enduring as I coordinated eye and ear procedures. I found that I could remember sound symbols longer, even permanently establish them in my mind-brain if I combined the singing of nonsense sounds with the "punching" technique I described in the previous chapter. It was necessary to begin slowly, singing a very slow song. How fast can one "punch"? Gradually, I would increase the pace and gradually my confidence would grow. Pictures and sounds of letters danced in my head to a silly song and punching hands. After these exercises, reading and writing letters and words was a whole lot easier.

Today I use procedures related to these, though much refined by experience, in working with learning-disabled children. Some of these procedures are described in Part Four of this book.

Auditory blending is an aspect of auditory perception that causes difficulty for many learning-disabled children. Let's use the word *blend* as an example. The child looks at it in confusion.

"*Sound it out,*" *says the teacher or parent.*

No response.

"*OK, I'll help you, 'bul-luh.' What comes next?*"

No response.

"*Buh-luh-eeh-nuh-duh,*" *says the adult.*

No response.

"*OK, I'll make it easier. Listen, will you! 'Bul-ulll-enn-duh.' Now say the word.*"

"*Bullfight.*"

"*OK.*" *(Adults use "OK" with these children so much because they hope things will someday be OK.)* "*OK. You got the 'bul.' Listen to the rest. 'Bul-ulll-enn-duh.' *"

"*Beautiful.*"

"*OK, but try again. You lost the beginning but some thinking must be going on between your ears. You're talking now. Go ahead. Try again. 'Bul-ulll . . .' *"

"*Bullshit.' Oh God. Did I say 'bullshit'? I'm sorry. It's the first thing that came to my mind. Sorry. No, I'm really sorry.*"

"*You know that it can't be that word. The word we're looking for ends in 'duh' and has 'enn' in the middle.*"

"*'Bull-duh.' 'Bull-enn-duh.' I know. There's a Belinda in my class.*"

"*OK. I quit.*"

I have learned not to require these children to "sound out" single letters. Divide words into as few sound groups as possible and teach the children to speak the words with melody, even sing them, so that variations in pitch and intensity help one sound group to "overflow" into the next. In doing this you utilize a strength common to many learning-disabled children. It appears in blending sounds and also in cursive writing as soon as they are able to form letters. The rhythmic, melodious muscle activity involved in this kind of writing blends well with melodious speech. The coordinated use of both is a powerful tool in teaching auditory blending as well as many other skills most useful to learning-disabled children. The concept of "melody" and its role in mastery of learning disability is extremely significant. I devote chapter 11 to an exploration of this concept.

I will use the final part of this chapter to discuss a function of the ear that has nothing to do with hearing. Inside the external ear, beyond the eardrum and the middle ear, behind and above the inner ear, lie three semicircular canals. These canals might be thought of as remnants of the primitive ear, throwbacks to early evolutionary ears when primitive creatures did not use ears for hearing but for balance. However, unlike another primitive anatomical remnant, the appendix, these canals are not useless. They continue to give the body its sense of balance. Each canal is filled with a fluid and contains sensory cells that end in hairs. These hairs respond to changes in the position of the body. As the head moves, the fluid moves also, pushing against the hair and registering any change in balance. The messages from these balance sensors go to a part of our brain called the cerebellum. In contrast to the cerebrum (our main brain), the cerebellum is small, one eighth the weight of the cerebrum. In fact *cerebellum* in Latin means "diminutive brain." The cerebellum resides just inside the nape of the neck. Like the cerebrum, it is divided into two hemispheres and contains both white and gray cells. Indeed, it is a second brain. But it is a brain that mind does not or cannot relate to. Its functions are autonomous, uninformed by mind and not informing mind. We might call it a primitive brain. The cerebellum has direct nerve lines to the semicircular canals of the inner ear. It is the center of balance for our body. Since we must maintain not only inner balance but balance in relation to the external world, the cerebellum receives nerve fibers from parts of the cerebrum that record what the eyes see and the ears hear. The cerebellum, then, is the center that coordinates vision, hearing, and muscle action so that we do not walk into telephone poles or fail to respond to the startle effect of a car horn. It controls our vertical and horizontal position in space.

For many years after I learned of the coordinating functions of the cerebellum and semicircular canals, I felt particularly enlightened regarding the cause of my learning problem. I was convinced that it was "hiding out" somewhere in a dark corner of my little second brain, an impairment causing me to misperceive the direction and sequence of letters in words — even to be unaware that some of the letters were there at all. The functions of the cerebellum are autonomous, automatic. This fact convinced me all the more that the culprit in my problem was my cerebellum, for I was never conscious of my misperceptions when I committed them and only occasionally afterward. Even as an adult, I couldn't always "see" the difference between words like cerebrum and cerebellum, unless I paid careful, self-conscious attention. I blamed this need for extra effort on the cerebellum. Also, my ability to use oral language as a child, adolescent, and young adult was stronger than that of many learning-disabled children that I later came to work with and know. Since my particular learning disability manifested itself more often as perceptual confusion than semantic confusion (though both were involved), I assumed that perceptual weakness caused any semantic difficulty I experienced. So I did not feel justified or inclined to blame my main brain in any way. Learning disability even in my early years of teaching was for me a dysfunction of inner ear and cerebellum, not perception and mind-brain.

I abandoned this belief almost twenty years ago. A blending of my personal and teaching experience eventually taught me that daily I was encountering a group of children who misperceived only when they had to relate meaningless symbols to meaning — a meaning once or twice or three times removed from the concrete world they knew as home. I was dealing with a semantic problem. I could no longer excuse my mind-brain or theirs either.

Some recent trends in learning-disability research and

treatment are placing strong emphasis on the inner ear/cerebellum connection. A few of these trends place the cause of learning disability and the entire treatment package for it — the whole ball of wax — squarely in this inner-ear/cerebellar function. When I read about these trends, I undergo a déjà vu experience. Feeling some nostalgia for the simpler, good old days, I want to advise, "Don't take this path. It only goes a short distance into the learning-disability maze, takes a few turns, then it ends."

Only recently the brain of a deceased dyslexic (*dyslexia* refers to a severe reading problem and is one of many manifestations of learning disability) underwent gross and microscopic anatomic analysis. The investigation revealed some peculiarities in cellular arrangement in the left hemisphere of the cortex.

A novel electroencephalographic (try this word for perceptual jitters) technique called the Brain Electrical Activity Mapping (BEAM) was used in a study of dyslexic and nondyslexic boys. The dyslexic group showed greater slow-wave activity in the left posterior hemisphere (an important semantic area) of the cortex.

Neither of these findings is clinically diagnostic, nor does either of them even begin to inform us about treatment. The findings do provide additional evidence, however, that in dealing with learning problems among our bright, normal population, we are dealing not just with eye, ear, gross and fine motor activity, or balance, but with the maze of connections that all of these have with mind and brain.

9

Hands and
the Mind-Brain

MANY YEARS AGO I watched while a photographer was taking school pictures of my SLD class. I noticed that the children were as self-conscious about their hands as they were about their smiles. Every adjustment of face, mouth, and head was accompanied by an adjustment of hands. I watched in fascination as a little girl brought her hand up to push back her hair and then didn't know what to do with it. As she positioned her hand at her side, on her lap, on top of her other hand, on her knee, and finally under her other hand, her face underwent a series of changes from smile, to frown, to scowl, to worry, and back to smile. Her hand seemed to be directing the performance as if it had a little mind of its own tucked into it.

I have observed repeatedly over the years that many learning-disabled children, when confronted with the "Draw-a-Person" body-image test, draw the hand completely out of proportion to the rest of the body — much too large, too prominent, sticking out at weird angles. Many begin the drawing with a hand and go on to the rest of the body from there. Here are a couple of recent examples.

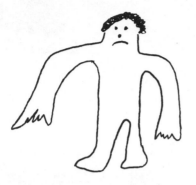 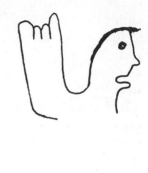

Anybody who has had dealings with SLD children knows that their hands are busy constantly — tapping and rolling pencils, stretching and winding rubber bands, bending and jabbing paper clips, picking at warts, scabs, and fingernails, scraping varnish off desks, wadding paper, shredding erasers, drumming on desk tops, scraping paint off pencils and splintering the pencil afterward, moving to the mouth so that blood can be sucked from real or imaginary wounds received during the foregoing activities. Have you ever noticed the almost hypnotic fascination that SLD children seem to have for small miscellaneous, hand-occupying objects? I learned early in my teaching career to hide rubber bands, paper clips, gummed stickers, staples, pins, thumbtacks, and string. I don't even allow paper and pencil within hands' reach until it is time to write. Then I make sure it's used for its purpose.

I have read that the area of the human brain allotted to the hand is unexpectedly large, equal to that allotted to face, mouth, and vocal organs and in proximity to it. It seems logical that the development of hands was, in part, linked to the development of communication in humans. How often have you seen a person gesture to enhance communication? The more tense the person becomes or the more engrossed in interpreting a deep or abstract thought, the more the hands pitch in to help communication flow. In my own experience with the phenomenon, I do not consciously invite my hands to join in; they seem to have a mind of their own and are gesturing wildly before I become aware of their movement and embarrassed when I see somebody staring at them instead of at my face.

In his book *The Man with the Shattered World*, Alexander Luria recalls his attempts to reteach a brain-injured war veteran how to read and spell. After failing with all the conventional methods, he chanced upon an extremely interesting phenomenon. One day, after almost despairing over teaching the young man how to recognize the word *tree*, he took the man's hand and started to force him to write the word. No sooner had the *t* been half formed than the man continued on his own, remembering and writing the whole of *tree* and saying, "t-r-e-e, tree." What his mind-brain couldn't remember his hand (or more correctly mind-brain-hand) could.

I had discovered years before reading this that many children (as well as adults) have hands that remember, hands that can tie eyes, ears, and voice together with mind for efficient learning. I also discovered that some children cannot easily integrate hand learning with mind learning. Their hands distract their minds. Like the adult who gestures so much he loses track of what he is saying, this kind of child will occupy his hands with so many disjointed activities that his mind becomes disjointed and unfocused. These children are our learning-disabled children. No wonder such youngsters make big ugly hands on their draw-a-persons, hands that seem to have a life of their own. Their own hands keep them in ugly, unlearning circumstances and seem to live apart from their minds and bodies.

I have found that in teaching the hands of an SLD child to cooperate and concentrate, I can teach his mind to concentrate. Chris, a boy of ten, gifted with above-average intelligence, had straight F's before I inherited him. His handwriting was imported from the twilight zone, one third printed, one third cursive, one third a combination of the two. For Chris, letters had no arbitrary shape or direction, lines did not exist, size was entirely subjective. The following is a sample of Chris's written interpretation of the word *smoke:*

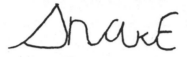

I recall staring at it in amazement.

"What's wrong?" asked Chris.

"You made a capital S," *I said.*

"That's a small s."

"Then why is it so big?"

"It's no bigger than the e."

"What about the m? *You made an* n."

"That's an m. *It has two humps. An* n *only has one. Like this."*

And Chris picked up his pencil and wrote:

"That looks like an r," *I said.*

"No, an r *is made like this."*

And he wrote:

R

"Well anyhow, that o *is a* u *for sure."*

"No, it's an o *all right. I make my* o's, a's, *and* u's *the same. It's easier."*

I wondered how much Chris's manual cop-out with these vowels contributed to another problem that he had — an inability to discriminate their sounds. I didn't wonder for long however. I began to experience that "hot collar" sensation that usually tells me when I've had enough. I took Chris's pencil and wrote the word *smoke* in cursive well enough to meet most arbitrary standards. Then I gave Chris his pencil and told him to write it very slowly below my *smoke.* I told him to really take his time, for this was the most important thing he had to do all day. He grabbed the pencil, bent his head all the way down to the desk (I'll discuss this phenomenon in a later chapter), screwed his face into a monumental parody of concentration, and duplicated my *smoke* beautifully. I told him to do it again. He did.

"Again," I said. He did.

"Again." He did.

"A little faster," I said. He wrote faster and lost little quality.

"Faster," I said. He did.

"Keep writing it faster each time," I said. He wrote it five more times. The last smoke *wasn't too much worse than the first.*

"Close your eyes and write it," I said.

"Impossible," he said.

"Do it," I demanded. "Start with your eyes open so that you start on the line, but close your eyes as soon as your hand moves." He did.

"Wow," he said.

"Do it again," I said. He did.

He wrote it six more times alternating between open and closed eyes. All attempts were good. I asked Chris to write the sentence, "The smoke got in his eyes." *Smoke* was beautiful. *The, got, in, his,* and *eyes* were from the twilight zone.

I asked Chris to read and was not surprised that his reading was like his writing. Receptive and expressive communication both relate to hands. He paused at unusual places; he modulated his voice at the wrong time; he read one word like an orator, and slurred the next like a wino. He coughed, he sighed, he scratched, he pointed to one word and read the next, he read one line twice and skipped the next one. He stopped often and asked "Where am I?" He assured me that he usually read better than this; he looked up and admitted that he really could not read very well. All the time his hands were going from a word, to his ear, to scratch his head, to scratch his ankle, back to a word, to wipe his eye, to pick his teeth, back to a word, to suck his finger as if he had injured it in reading (he told me it was an old injury that bothered him a lot). By the time he finished, he looked as if he had finished digging a deep ditch and I think he had expended as much energy.

I ordered Chris to keep his hands on his lap while he was reading. When he tried to move them, I held them there. He read a little better. I held his head straight with my hands. His reading improved a bit more.

Looking at the text he read, I asked Chris the simplest comprehension question I could think of. "What!" He almost shouted as if I had just touched him with a cattle prod. I asked him the question again. He had no idea what I was talking about. No miracles that day — just the very beginning of an important change for Chris.

This learning-disabled youngster became a good student within eight months, not special but in the mainstream. Over a period of time I trained his hands (I should say mind-brain-hands) to concentrate, remember, and join in rhythm with the rest of his person. This had much to do with his overcoming his learning disability.

It seems paradoxical that hands, which contribute to learning disability, can be used to enhance learning ability. Through the years, I have drawn three conclusions concerning the mind-brain-hand relationship that, I feel, are important if learning disability is to be mastered.

An essential function of the colossal and intricate network of ganglia that comprise the human central nervous system is to filter out and to edit internal and external impressions for the mind-brain. Without this editing service the unaware brain and aware mind would suffer an immediate monumental overload and would probably stop functioning on the spot. Imagine mind-brain-body trying to handle the full spectrum of infrared and ultraviolet light, the entire decibel range of pitch and intensity, the swing and sway of the thousands of little movements coming from its own proprioception, the full brunt of tactile sensation coming from every square millimeter of surface the body is touching, the groaning of its organs, the swishing of its blood, the rumbling of air in its lungs, the thunder of its own heartbeat.

Many learning-disabled children suffer from a much smaller overload. My guess is that these children overload their proprioceptive systems each time they try to read or write. Reading and writing require careful attention to the meaningless direction of visual symbols and the meaningless lines comprising these symbols. This attention is necessary so that these symbols can be coordinated with meaningless sound symbols, and strung together in meaningless sequences. After this is accomplished, a "Eureka!" of meaning is created. (Sometimes.) The child who is swinging one hand in every direction and nit-picking at this here and that there with the other (the very hands that should be constructing and remembering the direction and ordering of symbols) is sending an overload of direction to his mind-brain. The poor mind is trying to concentrate on an array of arbitrary directions while it is being flooded by flickers and flutters and spurts of more direction. It tells the central nervous system (in a subconscious way) that it cannot handle all this incoming nonsense. Obediently, the brain and nervous system kick the overload back into the hands, creating a cycle of distracting, unwanted movement.

Conclusion One: The learning-disabled person who learns to control his hands when he reads or writes, using them only for the writing task itself or to underscore only the most difficult words while reading, will concentrate better on the task at hand and perform better. During a reading exercise, a learning-disabled child should not point to words that he already can read. Nor should he do this with new words once he has learned them.

Most learning-disabled people do not use the same sequence in forming letters each time they write them, either in manuscript or cursive writing. For example, the child may use this sequence in printing a *b:*

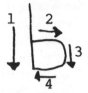

Another time he may use this sequence:

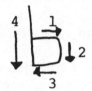

Another time this:

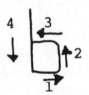

And so on. Sometimes he may start the long vertical line at the top; sometimes at the bottom. The appearance of the letter will often vary, depending upon the sequence used.

When the learning-disabled child forms his cursive letters in variant ways, he undermines the right directional flow and rhythm of cursive writing. The "goings back" and retracings he uses in writing words turn cursive writing into a cumbersome, inefficient tool. He tries to abandon it. If he is forced to use it, he often mixes it with manuscript writing in a futile attempt to make it more efficient for him.

When the mind-brain permits the child to express symbols in many variant sequences and forms, it is probably because it is receiving them with equal inconsistency.

Conclusion Two: The learning-disabled child must be taught to form letters and words with the same sequence of strokes every time he writes them. In this way, he will create an expressive efficiency that will improve his perception. Improved perception will make it easier for the mind-brain to synthesize percept and concept. Meaning surfaces more easily. The child gains in every way.

Most learning-disabled children draw concrete objects quite well. They are also adept at drawing random designs (much more complicated than letter writing) as long as the designs are not named. Many learning-disabled children can also move rhythmically as long as they are allowed to exercise free rhythm, unencumbered by instruction that divides a rhythmic pattern into parts.* These talents should be put to use. The learning-disabled child can learn cursive writing as an automatic rhythm and drawing exercise. Manuscript writing, requiring frequent pencil lifting and as many left-directed strokes as right, does not lend itself to rhythmic flow. Cursive writing does. And the learning-disabled child can learn how to do it. This ability can form the base for his semantic learning. Some procedures for learning the above are discussed in Part Four.

Conclusion Three: Teach cursive writing to a learning-disabled child at the earliest age possible. When he is able to print letters, he is also able to learn cursive writing.

---

*This does not contradict the fact that some learning-disabled children have coordination problems. When the child fits the definition of learning disability used in this book, the coordination problems are subtle more often than not. They usually manifest themselves in bilateral or directional confusion and become overt and disabling only in "instructional situations." Even here their disabling effect can be overcome.

10

Speech and the Mind-Brain

I REMEMBER Joey very clearly. He came into my life eleven years ago, when he was eleven, and left my life ten years ago. I didn't teach Joey in any formal class. I was a sort of supervisory teacher in SLD education that year. Joey was transferred from teacher to teacher during the year for three reasons. He couldn't read a word. He had a superior IQ. He seemed dedicated to using his IQ for a single purpose — driving teachers out of their profession. Joey was brought to me many times by teachers ready to self-destruct. I counseled Joey for a few minutes each time he showed up, but I didn't have any time to teach him. (I was having a brutally busy year.) Once I remember getting his mother in on the action, as any good supervisor should. I remember her coming into my room, sitting down, and sighing, as she said, "You can't tell me anything about Joey that I don't know. Talk, talk, talk. Move, move, move. He has always been so busy talking and moving that he hasn't discovered that a brain came with his body — not just arms, legs, and tongue."

Joey's mother and I didn't accomplish anything remarkable in our meeting, but her opening remarks (especially "Talk, talk, talk") occurred to me a few days later when Joey was dragged into my room again. "Do something with him or I quit," said his latest teacher. "Bang," said the door. "Sit down, Joey," said I.

Joey sat and said nothing for a change. He stared at me, lips trembling, for a few long moments, then the flood burst out.

"Let that old bag quit or fire her. She hates me and I hate her. Ask anyone, go ahead, ask anyone how she treats me. If you don't fire her, I'll tell my mom. That teacher's a old bitch."

This outburst was easy to remember. I wrote it down word for word just as he had said it. He knew what I was doing.

"You're going to put that in my file or show it to my mom," continued Joey, *"that doesn't scare me. You're a old bitch, too."*

Swallowing every ounce of pride I had, biting in my anger so hard that I almost popped a tooth cap inflicted on me the day before, I pushed the paper with the *written* outburst in front of him. "Read this," I demanded.

Joey looked at me as if I were not only an old bitch, but insane too. "I can't read," he said.

"Read it," I shouted, pounding my desk to relieve my anger.

"I don't know the first word," said Joey.

"Let," I said.

"What's the second?" he asked.

"I'll read you the first four words and then you'd better be able to read the rest," I said. "Let that old bag . . ." Joey took over and read the rest. When he finished, I was hoping he would jump up and down shouting, "I can read! I can read!" But Joey was no storybook person. He looked at me very blandly and said, "I really didn't read that because I just said it."

I decided to find time for Joey. I arranged to have him with me for one half hour each day. At first we went to a large room with a pair of walkie-talkies and talked to each other from different ends of the room. It was interesting to see Joey, in true SLD fashion, use the machine backwards, pushing the button to listen and releasing it to talk. Sometimes he would forget the button completely. He was having trouble coordinating communication and body rhythm, but it wasn't too long before he got the hang of it. This wasn't my purpose in using the walkie-talkies though. The messages we spoke were short and cryptic, easy to remember. And memory was enhanced by the manual use of equipment. We would go back to the office and I would ask Joey to repeat our conversation while I wrote it. He usually could. Then I would put the conversation in front of him in print and say, "Read this." He would read it beautifully but he always reminded me that, "This isn't really reading."

We followed this procedure every weekday for more than a month. Then one day Joey came in and announced, "I can read. Just write any paragraph and give it to me. Don't say it first." I wrote him a paragraph and he read it fluently. The paragraph contained second-grade-level vocabulary and Joey was in fifth grade, but what he did was "real reading." We coasted after that. Within another month, he was doing almost as well with fifth-grade paragraphs as with easier ones. Joey began to do much better in his regular classes and behaved better too. The only comment I heard from the teacher was, "Why didn't you do something sooner?"

I learned some important things from Joey. I learned that speech ties in more closely to reading than I ever imagined. My thoughts traveled to all of those SLD children I worked with in former years who spoke fluently and emphatically (though sometimes losing track of what they were saying) but read as if reading had absolutely no connection with communication or meaningful speech. The SLD child will read, "The boy fell from the tree and broke his neck" with the same expression and feeling as "How now brown cow."

I learned that fluency in speaking was not only valuable as a measure of improved reading skill, but even more valuable as a tool for teaching efficiency in reading. I learned that rhythm was most significant in this area; that rhythm in the mind-brain-voice apparatus could form the foundation and impulsion for rhythm in the audio-visual-mind apparatus necessary for reading easily.

Let us take a closer look at what I have come to call the Joey Factor. I have already stated in different ways that Specific Learning Disability is a condition that creates a gap between symbols and language.

Symbols do not confuse a child with a specific learning disability as long as the symbols themselves are concrete objects. This child has little trouble distinguishing symbols that do not relate to language and the meaning of language. He can cope with backgammon symbols, chess symbols, playing card symbols, electronic game symbols, and sport symbols.

It is when he must relate symbols to the meaning and concepts of language that he confuses them. The dysfunction involved in Specific Learning Disability lies in a gap between thought and spoken language, and between spoken language and the symbols that make it visual. The key to overcoming learning disability lies in bridging this gap.

A primary goal of any instructor of learning-disabled children must be to implement techniques that teach language expression and symbol usage in unity, constantly and intensively. Any method that falls short of this goal will probably disappoint the instructor and the child, and any improvement will fall below what should be established as the threshold of success.

Let's discuss here the Joey Factor as I use it with the learning-disabled child. The child in question cannot bridge the gap between the *symbols* of language and the *meaning* of language. I engage the child in conversation. He/she eventually says something personally meaningful. I write what the child says so that he/she can see it in symbolic language. I ask the child to read the words that I wrote. If the child reads the statement like a series of symbols devoid of meaning, I insist that it be read with the same expression and feeling with which it was originally spoken. Next, I require the child to write the statement *while saying it.* If, at first, the writing must be copied from my model, this is permitted as long as the child *says* the words while *writing* them. This is a cumbersome exercise at first. But I insist that the child write and speak the same thought simultaneously time after time, until speech and symbol blend in rhythm and unite in the wholeness of mind-brain-body.

When this happens, one strand of the symbol-meaning bridge has been built. What is left, perhaps, is the building of other strands; but this does not present a problem in planning, only in implementation. Repeat the procedure again and again with different language-symbol combinations culled from conversations, textbooks, and various assignments. Just be sure that meaning precedes practice and that speech accompanies writing. Work toward efficiency and speed. Don't worry about all the "information and concepts" that the child is supposed to be learning according to grade level and is missing. Build the language-symbol bridge firmly and securely. It may take many, many months. But when it is built, information and concepts can pass over it in caravans.

I have used speech as an instructional tool with learning-disabled children much more frequently after Joey than before Joey. It is rare that a student has reached Joey's level of competence so rapidly by using speech as a single tool. But the Joey Factor has added a dimension to my overall instruction procedure that, I feel, is very beneficial to any learning-disabled child who experiences it.

At least a few times every year teachers and other professionals who work with learning-disabled children ask me a variation of this question: "How can you place so much emphasis on speech as a remediative technique when many learning-disabled children are also language disabled?" An excellent question. Oral language deficits often accompany learning disability. In fact, oral language delay during pre-school years is a good predictor of future learning disability and school failure. Language deficits expose themselves through speech. Vocabulary may be limited, especially vocabulary expressing abstract notions through metaphor. Retrieval of known vocabulary from memory may be slow. Phonemes in words may be reversed or omitted or unnecessarily added or substituted. I have described this phenomenon already. Noun plurals, verb tenses, comparatives, negatives, and interrogative forms may be misused.

This is an excellent question indeed. I have often asked myself how speech can be such an effective instructional tool for so many learning-disabled children when for many of them it is a broken tool. Let me tell you some of the answers I have given to myself. They are satisfying to me, but they leave plenty of wide open space for mystery.

First, while many learning-disabled children are also language disabled, many are not. Many have little trouble grasping or expressing meaning apart from written symbols. Listen to them talk, argue, plead their case. Hear the neat, clever put-downs they dish out to classmates, brothers, sisters, or friends. See them size up the subtleties of any strife between teacher and class or between Mom and Dad, and take advantage of them. Watch them follow the plots of TV movies and remember every sequence in every film, while you're still trying to make some sense out of the one you saw three weeks ago. Feel intimidated as they outshine you in every mental game, verbal game (that doesn't involve spelling or reading), or puzzle that they can get their hands on. Feel stupid as they out-joke you, out-riddle you, and out-guess you.

These verbal learning-disabled children are generally those who have been able to establish a tenuous link between aural percept and semantic concept, but not between visual-aural percept and semantic concept. I say tenuous because in spite of their verbosity, these children will occasionally relapse into a reversal, omission, substitution, or addition. Or they will offend the ear with some outrageous syntax while not even trying to be "cool." I wonder if these relapses are due to faulty cross-indexing of multiple sensory experiences. As I mentioned already, none of our senses stands alone. I wouldn't be surprised if eye and mind-brain, with some help from muscle sense, were subverting ear and mind-brain.

Second, when the language that is used in speaking, reading, and writing practice is *conversational* speech, encouraged by the teacher but generated by the child, the language carries aural-semantic content; it already means something to the ear of the child. For this reason it is a viable tool, however underdeveloped it may be. The teacher can increase complexity (very patiently, very gradually) by reading selections from texts or books at the student's level, discussing them with much fanfare (every good teacher is an actor), and generating conversation from the contents. Once the student is drawn into the theater of language, don't let him escape. Like the comedian whose one joke leads to the next, the child, using some words, cuts a groove for further words. Also, just as the comedian is encouraged by an enthusiastic audience, so is the child encouraged by teachers and parents who become excited enough to "ham it up."

Third, in order to develop oral language the child must be aware of concrete reality, able to perceive it and manipulate it. Then he must match aural symbols with this reality and retain them. Then express them. In order to develop visual language he must add visual symbols to the above composite and retain them. Then express them. All of this, I feel, has evolved in mind-brain as a total package. Percept links to concept and concept to percept within each level and beyond each level to the next. The linkage binds early steps to late ones. Learning usually climbs up this latticework, but it can also climb down. Reading and writing can stimulate speech, just as speech can stimulate reading and writing. At least in my experience.

Let me conclude this chapter on a soapbox. It is my conviction that much *oral* work is essential to the academic and personal growth of learning-disabled children. (With these youngsters the personal depends so much on the academic.) For this reason, I feel that individualized reading programs are a disservice to learning-disabled children, at least until they develop reading fluency. Special teachers inherit a group of learning-disabled children with many levels of competency. They have been taught to individualize in the face of this challenge. So they must put each of their students into his own "special program." They do their best to get around to help each student, but the student can go for hours or even days without a chance to read out loud. They seldom if ever get the opportunity to speak, write, and read simultaneously. (Speaking and reading skills blend when the student speaks words as he writes them.) Parents approve of the individual approach because they think that individualization means individual help for their children. Can't you realize, teacher and parent, that frequent, intensive, daily, hourly oral reading and oral writing are essential to a learning-disabled child's growth? If you shove aside opportunities to blend speech rhythm with reading and writing rhythm you shove aside opportunities to use a most important tool in building reading, writing, spelling, and computing skills. You may not be able to build much of an academic structure without it.

If you were to chance into one of my SLD classes one weekday you probably wouldn't see children hunched over desks in individual carrels or solitary desks working at individual assignments. You would be more likely to see a bunch of children reciting the same paragraph over and over. You would also see a man who appears to be a middle-aged joker orchestrating this performance with his arms and voice to ensure fluency and expression. Then you would see him pass out paper containing the paragraph (sometimes missing desks and giving two to one student — not all the effects of SLD are overcome, just the worst ones) and listen to each student read the same words he was just reciting with the same fluency and expression. Individuals would read it, two or three would read it together, the class would read it in unison. You would probably hear some student comment, "I already know this stuff," and hear the teacher answer, "I know, but this will help you with the harder stuff. Just keep reading." And the student will.

After this you will see the students turn to individual assignments for a while. Some of these assignments seem strange. They involve reading and writing upside-down, reading and writing with books in front of mirrors, some walking and pacing, and strange but patterned hand and foot movements. One student is somehow using the square tiles on the floor to reinforce a word list he has. He leans in one direction, then another, still another, and finally settles on a particular tile. Then he sits down and writes something. Some students are working on regular textbook assignments. (The purpose of these exercises is explained in Part Four.)

Then the teacher begins a lesson in math. Everybody reads a word problem; then the teacher orchestrates the steps necessary to solve the problem. He makes the students say the steps without hesitation or doubt in their voices. Then they all do the problems together, saying each step and writing each step. The same complaint crops up: "I already know this." The same answer is given: "It will help you with harder stuff. Just do it." Another problem of the same type is done this way. Then another. After this, the students work individually on problems that duplicate the pattern of the problems that the class did in unison. They are able to handle this individual work with minimal help.

If you ask the teacher what he is doing he will answer, "I'm teaching a rhythm. The best way I know to teach reading or math to learning-disabled children is to incorporate into these disciplines the rhythm of speech." "He talks like a trainer, not a teacher," you think. Your assessment is accurate, in part. I am a trainer, but also a teacher.

Last year my son had a bad accident while he was riding his bike. He ran into a car (or the car ran into him). He broke his femur so cleanly that two thirds of his leg lay at a ninety degree angle from the rest of it. After months of traction and body casts, he began therapy. The therapist didn't teach the phenomenon of walking — the bones, muscles, tissues, and nerves involved. He simply exercised the necessary muscles and trained my son to walk again. "Move the bad leg as you move the good one," he said. And he made him do this over and over again. In my language, he was saying, "Take a rhythm you have and use it to learn a rhythm that you lost." He was "training" my son, but he knew that after the training this boy would learn to run again, to jump, and to play football.

I say to my learning-disabled students, in so many words, "Let's take a speech rhythm you have (whether fluent or not) and use it to learn a rhythm you don't have. With this rhythm, I'll train you how to read, write, spell, and compute. But I have something extra for you. I'll teach you to use these skills for thinking, planning, organizing, and creating. After this you'll be able to go into any class, anywhere, and learn with the best of them. Bear with me. It won't take as long as you think."

When a parent or teacher deals with a learning-disabled child, he or she is first of all a dedicated trainer, then a dedicated teacher. If this sounds harsh, enter the head of an SLD child and ask him what he wants more than anything. He will say, "To catch a big fish" or "To knock Harold's teeth down his throat." Don't give up. Get deeper into his head and you'll hear him saying, "I want to overcome this confusing mess that keeps me from being normal. Train me. Teach me. I don't care. Just do it. If you can't, then leave me alone."

I trained myself to overcome learning disability when I was a child. I had to. Nobody around me understood my handicap. Today there is plenty of understanding available to learning-disabled kids. There just isn't enough proper training.

11

Body Melody

THIS CHAPTER is about *melody*. I use this term in preference to *rhythm* because it describes better the coordination of ear and eye with body and mind-brain. In music, melody is a pattern of tones and rhythms producing a final product — a refrain or a song. In symbolic learning, melody patterns ear, eye, and mind-brain into a unified act of perception, making conception easier and producing the ability to link symbols with semantics.

Melody, as I use the word, does not refer to teaching through music, though the attempts of learning-disabled children to learn musical instruments contributed to my realization of its importance. Some years ago, a twelve-year-old student of mine named Sandra was taking piano lessons and getting nowhere. Her piano teacher meticulously taught her scales and a few chords from the beginner's book, but the child was unable to play even the first simple song the book presented. She became very discouraged and her mother was even more discouraged. I knew very little about music beyond knowing what I liked to hear and didn't like to hear, but an idea occurred to me. Why doesn't this child just learn a couple of songs, memorize them with mind and hands and ear, even if it takes twenty lessons? Forget about scales and chords and how they relate to piano keys. Just memorize the finger and

key movements and learn to play a couple of songs beautifully. The piano teacher was horrified when I suggested this,
so I located another teacher who was willing to give it a try.
It did take almost twenty lessons to the best of my recollection, but my student eventually played two songs beautifully
and confidently. At this point, I told her teacher to show her
how scales and chords and keys related to the songs she had
memorized. She learned this more quickly than anybody anticipated. She learned new songs rapidly, learned to read music, and soon became an excellent piano player. She was very
happy with herself. Her mother was ecstatic. I was curious.
How could I relate this music experience to reading and spelling, for Sandra was still very far from excellent in these
skills?

Another series of incidents with an SLD boy and his drums
brought back recollections of my "boom boom" days in kindergarten. Mark wanted to learn the drums so his parents,
who hoped that he would somehow learn something, brought
him a drum set and lessons to go with it. His efforts to learn
rhythm and cadence were disastrous. His nerves and his parents' and teacher's nerves became stretched as tight as the
drum. I made a suggestion to the parents. "Just let him pound
away," I told them. "Maybe he'll find some pattern of rhythm
inside himself that he can relate to the patterns in the lessons." They said that they would give it a try but would buy
earplugs. Several weeks later, they told me that their son was
learning how to play the drums.

A long, long time ago, before anybody thought of the label
SLD, dancing lessons were popular in school. The school
where I taught moved right with the times and incorporated
dancing in its program. I was teaching the class on the bottom rung of the "homogeneous grouping" ladder, so most of
my students were learning disabled by today's standards. The
dancing classes became such a source of embarrassment for
the kids and me that we connived to schedule field trips each
time our turn came around. The principal caught on to our

tactics and grounded us. My kids, forced to perform, were terrible. "One, two, three, four; one, two, three, four; faster, faster," sounded like the death march. We tripped; we collided; we froze and didn't move at all. Since we couldn't master the one, two, three, four, the teacher went on to the next lesson. "One, two, cha, cha, cha; one, two, cha, cha, cha." My God, what a disaster. My class looked as if it couldn't learn a single "cha" in thirty years, never mind three "chas" with a "one, two" in front of them. The teacher didn't help either. He was imported from outside the school and I could tell that he hated us. The happiest event of our school year was the time he went home with stomach cramps just before our turn was to begin. I empathized with my class. I knew that I would be just as "klutzy" as they were if I had to be up there dancing with them. I'm still a learning-disabled dancer. This can cause some harrowing moments when you're married to a cha-cha-ing, rhumba-ing, tango-ing Latin, as I am.

I decided to push aside the desks in my room, put a record on a borrowed phonograph, and let my students move to the music any way that they wanted to. They participated with gusto every time I did this. The other students and some teachers felt that this was all the proof they needed that we were "unwired." But the kids ignored all the heckling more easily than I did. You can guess the eventual outcome. After a few free-flow rhythmic sessions, the group started to perform better during the dance classes. They never became the best in the school, but they weren't embarrassed anymore — and the dance teacher didn't develop any more stomach cramps just before our turn.

Music and dance weren't the only contributors to my concept of melody. I often thought back to my long hours as a child struggling with a disability that I didn't understand but knew I must overcome. One thing from this period stuck in my mind, perhaps because I did it so often. I remember having so much trouble with individual words that I would memorize entire paragraphs to see how the words fitted together.

If this doesn't sound logical, let me explain. Do you remember those old spelling books in which the words you had to know were listed in a column on the left side of a page and contained in a paragraph on the right side? Well, I remember reading and then writing those paragraphs, time and time again until they blended with my hands and eyes and ears and body and became a part of me. I remember a slight improvement in my school performance, then a greater one; eventually I was functioning like everybody else. I remember getting so engrossed in these paragraphs as I improved in school that I would read them upside-down and sideways. This seemed to wipe away a lot of the perceptual cobwebs that I ran into every time I read. I would even write a word, then turn it upside-down, and using the upside-down word as a model, I would write the word upside-down. Eventually I could write words upside-down without the model. I made sure, in doing this, that the words were positioned correctly when I turned the paper right side up. I learned cursive writing in this manner too. It was more difficult, but when I gained skill, it was also more rhythmic. If you think this is an easy thing to do, try to write *try* upside-down, cursive and manuscript writing. Go ahead. Up becomes down, right becomes left, all relationships between symbols switch position. I think that if you do this upside-down stuff often enough and become fairly proficient at it, your mind-brain starts to dump out most of the perceptual garbage it has been carrying and begins to perceive with new and better awareness. I reached a point at which I could write whole lines upside-down and sideways, too:

Students can learn
to do this also.

(Students can learn to do this also.) It was as if something in my mind were telling me, "Look at these symbols, examine them from every angle, write them so you get to know them up close from every angle, build their 'melody of movement' into your body and mind-brain. You'll seldom confuse them again." As I began to feel comfortable and confident with the symbolic language of these paragraphs, I began to feel more comfortable with every other subject in school.

More than music, dance, and personal memories contributed to the development of my concept of melody. As I began to think about the relationships among various experiences that I had had in dealing with Specific Learning Disability, other tie-ins began to surface in my mind. After my children were born, I learned that babies didn't begin to speak with a single grunt but a series of rhythmic grunts — that when new sounds or words jumped out of my infants' vocal apparatus they seldom materialized alone; they were surrounded by other sounds and grunts and expostulations. If a sound or word materialized alone and lonely it repeated itself as if looking for company. "Da" was seldom just "Da." Most of the time it was "Da, Da, Da." A sense for language (and let me add to this the symbols that distill language to writing) seems to develop in a sort of linguistic rhythm that is probably learned from the environment but also seems to be built into a body-mind ready to receive.

These observations have been confirmed every time that I have tried to teach English grammar. It has usually been impossible for me to teach how the parts of language relate in a particular sentence until my students have become very familiar with the rhythm of that sentence. I require them to read the sentence many times until they settle on a rhythm that is comfortable and meaningful to them.

Have you ever noticed that a fifth-grade SLD student reads with fluency similar to that of a first-grade beginner although he can read far more words? Instead of reading, "The boy tripped over a root in the sidewalk," in the same flowing way that he would say it in conversation, he reads, "Thee boy tripped over A root in Thee sidewalk." I require him to read the sentence as he would say it, rhythmically, and then to write it rhythmically, without pausing at inappropriate junctures and without going backward with frequent erasures. If he makes a mistake, he goes on and corrects it in the next writing. I never permit him to pause in the middle of a word (after initial practice) while either saying or writing the sentence. After he has written the sentence a few times, I require him to write it again (just as rhythmically) with his eyes closed. He continues to write it, one time eyes open, one time eyes closed, until the sentence melds into his mind-body. When this happens, he shows a readiness to understand grammar when I teach it. For SLD children, it seems that practice in fluency must precede fluency in practice.

I've saved until now my best example of melody. Travis, age eleven, was a superb natural athlete. As I recollect, he could outrun, outjump, outflip, outthrow, outcatch, outshoot, outhit, outskate, outblock, and outmaneuver any preadolescent I can remember. His agility, in my estimation, was extraordinary. Yet Travis could barely read, definitely could not spell, could not memorize addition or multiplication tables, and was the unproud possessor of a most bizarre, illegible handwriting (worse even than Chris's!).

Learning-disability literature in the early 1960s placed much emphasis on physical coordination delays and problems for diagnosis and much emphasis on perceptual motor training for remediation. Travis's mother (like many other mothers of learning-disabled children) was familiar with some of this literature and because of this familiarity could not accept the fact that her son had a learning disability. I remember a conference with Travis and his mother that followed these lines.

MOTHER: Travis cannot be learning disabled. He's been well coordinated since he could walk. Our whole family are good athletes. Blame his problem on his teachers. They didn't know how to teach.

LYMAN: I'm sure many students learned from them.

MOTHER: Well, they didn't know how to teach Travis.

TRAVIS: Mom, it wasn't the teachers' fault.

MOTHER: Well, it's certainly not my fault or yours.

LYMAN: It's nobody's fault.

MOTHER: It has to be somebody's fault.

LYMAN: Can't something just happen to be a certain way without anybody's being responsible?

TRAVIS: Yeah, Mom, it's just the way I am. Nobody's to blame.

MOTHER: You're not the way you are. And somebody is to blame.

TRAVIS: I'm just slow.

MOTHER: If you say that again, I'll hit you right here in front of Mr. Lyman.

TRAVIS: Here we go again.

MOTHER: You keep your mouth closed. If you open it again, I'll knock some sense into you. That's more than your teachers did.

LYMAN: Look, let's forget the past. Travis seems bright enough. Let me do my best and we'll see what happens.

MOTHER: Good luck. I hope you do better than those other hopeless teachers.

I was fortunate enough to have great success with Travis. I transferred his body-mind-brain melody for athletics to perceptual, semantic melody, his physical coordination to sensory coordination. This is an excellent kind of transfer, because skill in one area is not lessened in transfer; it merely spreads out to incorporate the new area. Travis, already well coordinated, steamed through my "melody" techniques with speed, grace, and precision. His ability to compete in the semantic world increased rapidly. He became much more proud of his academic growth than of Little League trophies and ribbons.

Now that I've given this background, I'm ready to define my kind of *melody*.

Abstractly and poetically, melody is that center of wholeness in a frog that makes it jump, in a lizard that makes it skitter, in a dog that makes it fetch, in a bird that makes it fly, in a human that makes it communicate with spoken and written symbols. Without melody (ease at being what we are and doing what we do), we move without direction, we see and hear without perceiving. The person without semantic melody is, in a very real way, separated from his species. This is the lot of the SLD child. If he remains separated he can hurt the species. (Consider the prison statistics I mentioned earlier.) If he finds in himself the melody essential to symbolic communication he joins the species and makes it healthier. (Consider Albert Einstein, Woodrow Wilson, Thomas Edison, William Butler Yeats, Hans Christian Andersen, and many others who would probably be considered learning disabled if judged by today's standards.)

Concretely and pragmatically, what I call melody is a pattern of rhythmic movement developed in the mind-brain-body as it coordinates with the eyes and ears during the process of learning and communication. This pattern is externalized in the hand as we write (especially during cursive writing); in the musculature of the vocal apparatus as we speak and read; in the movement of the eyes as we read and write; in the apparatus of the ear as we hear, speak, and engage in internal hearing when we read and write; in the cerebellum and inner ear as we apply direction, balance, and consistency to our reading and writing. Melody facilitates the whole learning and communication process for us.

We all develop our individual, personal melodies. If we didn't we would all have identical handwriting and would speak and read with the same inflections, pauses, and speed.

Most children seem to have developed their personal melody naturally. Nobody taught it to them. They developed it in their early attempts at movement and speaking and later in their first attempts at reading and writing. Soon they perfected it to the point that it became their greatest ally in future learning.

Learning-disabled children are those who never developed this melody. Melody, in my opinion, is almost essential to the learning-disabled child's success. Why? Especially since learning disability is in great part a semantic disability? I can understand how melody can have a positive influence on perception, but I cannot understand how it influences symbolic concept formation — and percept must unite with concept if learning disability is to be mastered; yet we can all see it happening. I can only conjecture about this. Join me in conjecturing.

Melody creates a perfect composite in all areas of perception that I discussed earlier. It ties together present and past sensory impressions, for body-mind-brain remembers rhythms. Walking, swimming, dancing (once learned) are not forgotten.

Melody by definition is a composite of total sensory input. No sense can stand alone when melody is at work. When body-mind-brain dance to melody there are no wallflowers (or as my learning-disabled daughter used to call them, "no flowerwalls").

Melody unites reception and expression. It is a single act of input and feedback. When my feet tell mind-brain that they're going to dance, or my hand says it's going to write, the feet are dancing and the hand is writing almost without mind awareness. Input overflows into feedback. If melody is involved, eyes, ears, and the rest of the body have no choice but to join in.

Through melody, the learning-disabled child establishes fluid balance while perceiving, with senses cooperating instead of warring. A person blind from birth who receives sight cannot handle the display of color and form his eyes receive.

For weeks or longer he must close them in order to reestablish sensory balance. The learning-disabled child, in my opinion, acts in a similar way. He must block the rush of one or more senses to balance the rest. This is especially true when he must engage in "symbolic learning." Symbols are difficult for him, so his mind-brain calls forth reinforcement through almost every sensory avenue. The onrush is too great. Melody establishes the balance he needs.

But where does this leave the composite of percept and concept? When the learning-disabled child reads or writes with melody, his mind-brain receives a total symbolic percept. It does not get a hint from the eyes, a hint from the ears, a hint from the body sense, a hint from kinesthesia, a hint from speech, a hint from visual memory, a hint from auditory memory, a hint from body memory, a hint from tactile memory — one hint at a time and often in conflict. It receives all of these hints at once. Many hints given at once almost give away the meaning of a riddle. Perhaps the mind-brain of the learning-disabled child merely makes a low-risk guess or doesn't have to guess at all with the flood of connected hints that melody provides. For the learning-disabled child who practices melody, as I have defined it, is right most of the time.

Let's compare the percept-concept composite of those not learning disabled, to a puzzle. The pieces are the percept; the completed puzzle the concept. Semantic meaning is assured with the completion of each puzzle. Melody presents a puzzle to mind-brain, completed instantly. Semantic success is assured.

The learning-disabled child is not so fortunate. But a good guess, backed up by strong clues woven together by melody, is almost equal to certainty. This "almost equal" gives the learning-disabled child enough support to master semantics.

12

Attention, Memory, and the Mind-Brain

ATTENTION. Ah, there's the rub. "If he could only learn to pay attention, then he would learn everything else." No symptom of learning disability short of reading failure is mentioned more frequently than inattention.

The school records of a learning-disabled child speak of inattention from first grade on. Parents complain and worry about complaints of inattention at school and are confused about inattention at home. "He can watch TV or tinker with something for hours without distraction, but try to help him with homework or give him some small responsibility around the house and he skitters like a butterfly one moment and skids to a halt like a donkey the next."

Pediatric neurologists have raised chronic inattention to the status of a syndrome, ADD (Attention Deficit Disorder).

Adults responsible for the attention of a learning-disabled child and his concomitant growth in learning have three choices. Choice one: Train the child to pay attention. Choice two: Compete with TV. Become a personality — comedian, circus performer, Sesame Street actor, and big city detective. But be careful. The child probably will pay attention to you for a while and then switch to another channel. Choice three: Tinker along with him all day. The problem here is that he doesn't meet his responsibilities and you don't meet yours. I recommend choice one with interludes of two and three when the going gets tense or tough.

The learning-disabled child becomes inattentive when he is required to apply himself to symbol-semantic tasks or to organizational, temporal schemes. His mind-brain is not fine-tuned to these two requirements and he gets fuzzy signals in their presence.

How do we fine-tune the learning-disabled child? The technique is not the same for teaching symbols as it is for teaching concrete, organizational responsibilities. Both share two common areas, however. First, in either case it is important that the adult use words sparingly. Directions must be succinct. The child cannot filter too many words for they create interference. Second, when using these few words the adult should make sure that the child attends to them. He *can attend* if the words are few enough. Every time the child is allowed *not* to attend, he is learning inattention rather than attention.

The best way to teach the learning-disabled child organizational, temporal responsibility (take out the trash; make your bed; pick up your clothes; erase the board; clear your desk) is concrete demonstration. If he is shown how to do the required tasks, if the adult does them with him for a while, he will learn to do the tasks and not just tinker with them or ignore them. If the child is shown when to do the task, if the adult does them with him at that time for a while (as soon as you get up; after breakfast; when the bell rings; when I give you this signal; after lunch; as soon as you get home from school; after supper; before bed), he will learn to do the tasks at that time rather than ignore them or overlook them.

The best way to teach this child to attend to symbol-semantic tasks is by use of written and spoken language. In this abstract world, the child must be taught to *look at* rather than just *see*. *Looking at* is active, requiring a mind-brain decision to "draw inside" symbolic, visual images. *Seeing* is passive and does not require attention.

The child must also be trained to *listen to*, not just to *hear*. Like *looking at*, *listening to* is active. It, too, requires a mind-brain that is ready and able to "draw inside" symbolic sound. *Hearing* is passive, requiring no attention.

Finally, the child must be taught to "feel" inwardly the ups and downs and lefts and rights of letters and numbers, as well as experiencing them externally. In other words, kinesthetic touching and tracing exercises will not serve their purpose well unless the brain relates these exercises to inner messages of position in space provided by the body's proprioception. Herein lies the value of perceptual motor training when the movement involved duplicates the directions used in constructing letters.

A learning-disabled child who learns to pay attention usually reveals a remarkable short-term memory. He can often duplicate a series of simple visual designs better than most children can, if he can start duplicating right after they are removed from sight. He can often repeat a series of digits or words better than many others can, if he can start right after they are said. But make him wait a moment, stand up and sit down, circle his desk, shut the door, converse for a moment before starting, and his memory becomes dim. As one youngster told me after coming back from shutting the door, "I knew what you asked a minute ago, but you made the light go out."

Can the learning-disabled child develop long-term memory for abstract semantic symbols? This is a crucial question. If he cannot, he will never master his handicap and must cope in a literate society with "cover-up," anxiety, and perhaps rebellion. If he can develop such a memory, he will be able to master his handicap and live his life rather than cope with it.

My answer to this question is yes, but much hard work is required. This is no terrain for quitters, either adult or child. I hear that some people knowledgeable in this field say that the learning-disabled child can develop his long-term memory only minimally. Therefore, he will never read or spell "normally." I cannot agree with this. Long-term memory became my biggest weapon in mastering my handicap.

For many centuries it was felt that mind-brain with its memory component was like a muscle — if you exercised it enough, it became bigger, healthier, and more efficient. When I was young, most college-bound high school students were forced to study Latin. They were told that this study was good exercise for their brains and memories. With enough study of Latin, they would be able to learn practical disciplines more efficiently. Today, the analogy of memory and muscle causes chuckles of amusement at the innocence and simplicity of former educational and psychological theory. Today, most students of cognitive psychology believe that memory is physically determined. Individual differences allow for some small improvement, but generally a good memory remains good and a poor memory remains poor. Not much hope for the learning disabled here.

However, some modern researchers feel that memory can improve dramatically with training. (They studiously avoid using the muscle analogy or the word *exercise*. Who wants to be laughed at?) I'll join this second team if teachers are allowed to join. I feel that the learning-disabled child can be trained to remember symbolic language competently both over the short and the long term. I suggest a five-step process.

1. Train attention. Short-term memory follows.
2. Establish a basic outline of symbols. Make sure the child becomes very familiar with the outline.
3. Provide opportunities for linkage within each item of the outline and among the items. The more linkage provided, the better for the child.
4. Practice. Use a small segment of the outline to start. Then add on until the entire outline is memorized.
5. Incorporate the outline into the memory.

Step One was discussed earlier in this chapter. *Step Two* can be accomplished by many methods. Let me describe the method I use. After the child has learned the alphabet (techniques for this are discussed in Part Four), I select the short vowel *a* and pair it with each consonant in sequence. I say and write *ab* and ask for a word with *ab* in it. The student may respond "cab." I say and write his word after *ab*.

ab   cab

I continue with the rest of the consonants.

ac   act
ad   bad
af   after
ag   bag
ah   (no word for *ah*)
aj   (no word for *aj*)
ak   (no word for *ak*)
al   pal
am   camel
an   panel
ap   gap
aq   aqua
ar   arrow
as   ask
at   at
av   average
aw   (no word for *aw*)
ax   tax
ay   (no word for *ay*)
az   hazard

I erase the words and repeat the list again and again and again. The students say the words, then write them, then say and write them simultaneously to build familiarity. I also use a technique that coordinates visualizing, auditorializing (internalizing the sounds of the words), and proprioceptualizing (feeling the words in the muscles and joints). Since I am more interested here in giving an overview of my memory scheme, I will save an explanation of the above technique for Part Four.

When the student has achieved familiarity with the outline, he has already made use of *Step Three*, a step that requires multiple memory linkages. The learning-disabled child must have ample links available to him in order to establish a network of relationships. This network will provide sufficient back-up when he attempts to recall. If one link fails him, there are others. With this method, the child has a semantic link: he provided the words and knows their meaning. He has a phonetic link: he has already related the sounds to the words. He has a visual link: he related the letters to the sounds. He has an alphabetizing link: he knows that the consonants follow in sequence. He has two starting links, visual and auditory: all phonemes begin with the letter *a* and the sound "a."

In *Step Four*, the learning-disabled student practices saying and writing the first four words in the outline from memory. Short-term memory reaches saturation quickly, and four is generally his maximum. He practices these four again and again. Then he practices the next four, eventually saying and writing the first eight. After this he adds four more and continues the process until he can say and write the entire outline.

In *Step Five*, the student is required to recall the words out of order. I say, "Write your *ag* word, your *ad* word, your *as* word," and so forth. Or I will require the student to write and say the list backward or start at some point near the middle. When the student demonstrates effortless recall in doing the above, he has incorporated these words into his memory. They are there for the long term.

Much hard work has been required, but we have only begun. The student must assimilate all short vowels and short vowel variants in like fashion. Then he must make all long vowels and long vowel variants part of his memory. Next come consonant blends plus vowel, and depending on age, unpatterned vowel combinations, two-syllable words requiring the long vowel or doubling rule, prefixes and suffixes, even schwas. Finally, he must practice assimilation by recalling words from one group to the next.

A mountain of hard work! A mountain of time! But surmountable. I have little doubt that learning-disabled children can gain long-term memory for symbolic language. Like the mountain climbers, he must want the peak badly enough and so must his teacher. Success and victory make it all worthwhile.

Is this success among the ranks of the learning-disabled surprising to you? It isn't to me. There is a kind of child, surprisingly prevalent in the learning-disabled population, who develops and maintains a deep interest in a single category — inanimate or animate, current or past. These categories range from car models, planes, engines, and electrical components to insects, fish, and dinosaurs.

Almost every year, I have had the opportunity to teach one or more of these children. I don't have to go beyond the first week of school to discover that Harry is an "engine child" or that Robert is a "dinosaur child." Such children start early in the year and never let up. One tries to convert every class activity or discussion to an "engine activity" or a discussion of engines. The other tries to do the same with dinosaurs. The rest of the students show acute interest for the first few weeks of school, but after that:

"Mr. Lyman, if he says one more word about dinosaurs, I'll pull his tongue out and mount it!"

"You'd better make Harry shut up, Mr. Lyman, before I find an engine and cream him with it."

"Shut up, Robert."

"Shut up, Harry."

"Shut up, Harry and Robert."

"Shut up!"

"Shut up!"

This kind of child is shut up more times in a month than most of us in a lifetime.

Yet the remarkable thing about this child is that he can name, read, and spell (some errors here) almost every member of his chosen genre in spite of his learning disability. Try some of those dinosaur names. Quite a memory feat! This learning-disabled child seeks out reality, past or present. When he settles on a particular area of high interest to him, he remembers everything in that area, symbols and all.

I asked a "fish child" once how he remembered all those names. Not just easy ones like bass, trout, dolphin, and bluegill, but crevalle jack, buffalo fish, black crappie, and muskellunge.

"When you think about fish as much as I do, you'll remember them," he said.

"Usually I go by the first letters. When I think of a fish that begins with b *a whole bunch of them come to mind. I go fishing a lot too."*

Two interesting points in this answer: One, the "fish child" used linkage to help him remember. Two, he had developed a healthy blending of semantics and reality. "When you think about fish as much as I do . . . I go fishing a lot too."

Interference with the Mind-Brain

There once was a child named Clout
Who passed her young life in doubt.
Scenes passing by,
Sounds from the sky,
Which if any of these should she block out?

AS THE YEARS have rolled or staggered by (some years roll and some stagger in my profession), I have kept a log of my most successful experiences and my most successful failures (the ones that taught me something). I have also recorded memories of many of my most interesting students. Occasionally I have immortalized (???) a student in verse. Clout is one of these students.

Clout's actual name is Bridget. The boys in class called her Clout because she could hit a ball farther than any of them. The girls called her Clout also; at least the ones who wanted to be popular with the boys. Bridget loved this new name and used to sign her papers Clout (or sometimes Cout, or Klot, or Clot, or Clut, or Clote). I taught her when she was age eleven. She was one of the most distractable youngsters that I have ever worked with. In class, she could inhibit (block out) almost nothing. Every sight, every sound, every position and movement of her body distracted her. She is the only student

I remember who was distracted by her own voice. Sometimes Bridget would say a word and stop, startled by the sound of it. She was perpetual swivel, perpetual head jerk, perpetual bend over, perpetual lean over, perpetual motion. And she was hardly aware of her movement. Once, when Bridget had a foot under an adjacent desk, her head bent almost to the floor (apparently looking for the source of a noise beneath and behind her), the other foot pointing almost vertically at the ceiling, and her hands scratching her knees, I shouted in exasperation, "Bridget, pay attention." She swung her face forward, almost hitting her chin, and answered from the floor, "What?"

"I said, pay attention."

"Huh?"

"Pay attention."

"I am paying attention" (with much hurt in her voice).

"Not to me, you're not."

"I'm looking right at you."

"But you weren't before. Sit up and listen."

She sat up. "I'm paying attention."

"Good," I said, and resumed the lesson.

Before the third word was out my mouth, Bridget had taken approximately the same position as before, except her head tilted more to the left. Apparently the elusive sound had shifted. Her knees still itched.

Not many learning-disabled children inhibit as poorly as Bridget did, or block out as poorly as Clout. (I'm on a run here; had I thought of this eighteen years ago, I could have immortalized Bridget with two limericks!

> *There once was a child named Bridget,*
> *From morning to night she would fidget.)*

But most suffer from a level of distraction that interferes with learning.

Since I had to "work through" large amounts of distract-
ability every weekday, it became important to construct a
model that would work in dealing with it. I found that lack
of inhibitory skills (I'll call this disinhibition) had two close
relatives, impulsiveness and compulsiveness, and they too became part of my model. The model has served me well, so I
present it for your consideration.

The brain of the learning-disabled child is overloaded by
four kinds of input. *Input one* is the confusion, the try and try
again, presented to the brain by faulty perception.

Input two is the overabundance of input reaching the brain
from the muscles and joints of the body. Just as you occasionally call up body reinforcements to assist you when symbolic
learning becomes especially difficult (you squint your eyes,
bounce your knee, point at words, get up and walk around),
the learning-disabled child does likewise. Unlike you, however, he/she finds symbolic learning difficult constantly. So
the brain receives steady bombardment from the muscle
sense, not occasional nudging.

Input three has its source in the emotional tension generated by continuous fear of failure. This tension sends urgent,
severe alarm signals to the brain.

Input four is caused by physical discomforts, physical ten-
sions (from pain to itch to restlessness), which in turn are
caused by the emotional tension.

The brain, overwhelmed by such a flood, is unable to perform its usual filtering function and kicks many of these inputs back into the muscle and tissue neurons of the body,
including the neurons of the eyes, ears, and vocal apparatus. The body and its sensory systems are in turn overwhelmed. Trying to collate feedback and input, the child
becomes like the disoriented hunter who, responding to
every sound, shape, color, and movement, fires off in every
direction.

Enter mind. The child, urged by parent, teacher, peers, and

his own discomfort, seeks a solution. He may choose to short-circuit both input and feedback systems, reducing input to a mere trickle. He withdraws. During school hours, he wears a mask of "learned stupidity." If his withdrawal is severe, everybody worries about him. He is labeled hypoactive and sent for psychological and neurological tests. Only a very small percentage of learning-disabled children fit this category.

Most learning-disabled children use a different coping strategy — impulsiveness. Faced with a stream of sensory stimuli (internal and external), they focus on the first or most intense or most interesting — but not for long. The stream keeps moving and there are new firsts, new intensities, new interests. These children adopt a butterfly approach to learning and to life. They flitter from this first stimulus to this intense one, to this interesting one, to this new one. If the degree of impulsiveness is mild, they are called immature. If it is moderate, they are called overactive. If it is extreme, they are called hyperactive and medicated. "Hey, Mr. Lyman," they tell me when I first meet them, "I take hyper-pills."

Sometimes, a learning-disabled child will fixate on a particular pattern of stimuli that engages his interest or provides him refuge and will stay with it, repeating the same act over and over. The name for such activity is perseveration. I have seen learning-disabled children fixate on a particular kind of math problem they have learned and do page after page of the same problem — then insist on more. I have seen them fixate on drawing a single object (airplane, Snoopy, rocket ship, peace sign, smiley face) and draw it one hundred times a day. Day after day. When the teacher tries to wrench their attention from the fixation to learning, they strongly resent this invasion of their private, secure, pleasant world — because they know they are being forced back into a world of confusion, discomfort, and insecurity where impulsiveness is beyond their control. These are the children who have turned *im*pulsion into *com*pulsion. During preadolescence, they are few in number. During adolescence, they are legion.

I am only conjecturing when I say that the impulsive child can no longer tolerate his random approach to life as he reaches adolescence. Perhaps increasing social pressure, peer pressure, or home pressure forces him to face up to his impulsive behavior. This kind of behavior is tolerated in children because it comes across as immature and hardly anyone is surprised when a child acts immaturely. When the child reaches adolescence, this behavior is no longer immature. It has become inappropriate and unbearable. Under such pressures, it seems that the learning-disabled child tries to control his impulsivity and finds it impossible to do, so he fixates his attention on the first influence that can engage his interest, offer him acceptance, and provide him escape.

Unfortunately for the learning-disabled adolescent (and for his family and society), he often fixates on an experience with drugs and/or alcohol or an experience with engines, noise, speed, and the thrill of controlled power. If he can't control himself, he hopes he can at least control his motorcycle or fast car.

The learning-disabled person climbs the ladder from impulsive child to compulsive adolescent to disillusioned adult — unless he destroys himself along the way. This may seem melodramatic to you, but I've seen it happen often enough to know it's real. If my conjectures seem far-fetched, my observations are not. Impulsive learning-disabled children do become compulsive adolescents, and this is a shame.

So ends my model. What has it taught me? I have learned to play educational dominoes. I start by training "attention." When I train a child to pay attention, perception improves. When perception improves, "word thinking" improves. When word thinking improves, concentration improves. When concentration improves, emotional tension is relieved. When emotional tension is relieved, physical tension is lessened. Disinhibition falls, impulsion falls, compulsion falls.

The younger the child, the better the chance for success. The game of educational dominoes does the job best at the stage of inhibition, worst at the stage of compulsion.

14

The Emotions and the Mind-Brain

I'M GOING TO TAKE YOU for a ten-minute visit to a typical SLD class in Most Anywhere, U.S.A. We open the door to the classroom and there is a tremendous shuffle of desks as ten heads, necks, and torsos swing in our direction and then swing back as if controlled by a network of inner springs. You accidentally scrape your chair as you sit down and the heads, necks, and torsos swing again. You feel a little self-conscious. Why don't these children just shift their eyes in your direction or turn their heads a little? Why all this unnecessary movement and commotion? I suggest that you ignore any teaching that is going on and observe only the children. The hand antics that I described to you earlier are in progress. Foot tapping and shuffling is continuous. Occasionally a desk is pushed back to a wall and a child leans back. The culprit is told to put the desk flat so he doesn't mark the wall. He complies. Before twenty seconds pass, his chair is back against the wall and two cronies have joined him there. You get the impression that they are being more impulsive than disobedient. One child that you pick for special observation is leaning his head on one hand, then shifts it to the other hand, stops for a while, rolls up the corner of his paper with one hand, writes and erases with the other, writes and erases again until he erases a hole in his paper. He curses at the hole, three students laugh at him; he curses at the students and goes back to leaning his head on his hand.

Your attention shifts to another child. The teacher is leaning over him, helping him with an assignment. She puts an encouraging hand on his shoulder. The shoulder shrinks back from her touch as if it is sore and the child shifts his desk to avoid further touch. In general, there is much laughter going on (mostly the children laughing at each other), some whining, some complaining, ten faces furrowed in painful attempts at concentration — but no smiling, no relaxation, little enjoyment of the task at hand or of each other.

The atmosphere is tense, not because the teacher has created a tense atmosphere but because each child appears to carry his own tension — almost to the point of physical discomfort. You end your ten-minute visit feeling a little tense yourself — and more than a little depressed.

Each learning-disabled child lives in a teetering social structure, one that could collapse in on him at any moment. And he knows this. He knows that at school he must face up to an encounter with symbols and semantics in front of an audience (fellow students) and a team of judges (administrators, teachers, counselors, deans). He knows that he is called to this encounter daily, hourly, every minute. No escape from worry, fear, embarrassment, frustration, tears, and anger. No escape from any of these, for he experiences them all mixed together. Failures come too fast for him to organize and analyze feelings. There is too much garbled emotion. It cannot be filtered by his brain — or mind.

Often his audience turns judge. "Stupid, retard, low life." It is no help that he is placed with other learning-disabled children. Do unto others as has been done unto you. His classmates are the meanest of the mean. He must divert attention. Should he clown? Or "put down" someone else (put him down lower than himself), withdraw and refuse to participate, or knock over a desk, curse at peers and teacher, and create an interesting crisis for the school and himself? Or should he sit quietly and take abuse, blaming himself? He fears blaming himself. Each time he does this there is less left of him. Someday he might erase himself. On that day, he feels that he won't be responsible for his actions.

At home, the social structure also teeters. In his home he feels too much at home or not at home at all. Here, heaving his sigh of relief at the end of the school day, he lets all of his frustration, impulsiveness, disorganization hang out. Where can you do this if not at home? The family reacts to his demands and insouciance as you would expect them to react. Lectures, preachments about attitude, nagging, shouts, regretted name calling. He becomes the "family problem." And, in accordance with Murphy's Law, he gets worse. "Home, Sweet Home" becomes "Home, Bitter Home." Home just doesn't feel like home for him.

The learning-disabled child is a "normal" person who cannot perform "normally." A bright person who seems dull. How do his brain and mind handle this paradox? I think the brain does its equivalent of flashing an emergency light. "Stop! An emotion-laden paradox on top of the perceptual confusion this body keeps sending me. It's too much." The brain feeds it back to the body in the form of physical tension. Many learning-disabled children are physically tense people. And chronic physical tension can have severe consequences. Some therapists claim that the body's myofascial system (the connective tissue that supports and provides cohesiveness and fluid exchange for the musculoskeletal system) loses its elasticity when burdened by continual physical tension. Some go so far as to claim that muscles shorten and thicken; that connective tissue joins adjacent fascial envelopes and makes an unresponsive mass out of muscles.

Recent research shows some evidence that even fascial sutures in the cranium tighten, causing some restriction in the flow of cerebrospinal fluid.

I have observed over a long period that learning-disabled children are generally uncomfortable children, physically as well as emotionally. They are not at ease in their bodies. Many develop a postural set, a style of restricted movement. Head and limb movement is rapid, jerky, and irregular. Sometimes the head, shoulders, or hips develop a chronic lean. A few children develop curvatures of the spine. Rhythm is lacking in bilateral movement (movement that involves the right and left side of the body, such as walking, where the left arm swings while the right foot steps). The gait is strange; the arms swing too much or not enough; the feet shuffle too much or too little, giving a "Raggedy Ann" or "tin soldier" appearance. These children seem to be locked into a chronic dis-ease situation. Free emotional and physical flow seem impossible.

I hadn't been teaching SLD children long before I realized that I couldn't shout, threaten, push, pull, or yank them into learning. Each time I tried, I felt as if I were short-circuiting wires with no insulation. I learned that I couldn't even pat their backs in congratulation or praise without causing discomfort. I found that I couldn't use my hands, however gently, to turn their heads to face a worksheet or text without the same short-circuit.

On the positive side, I learned that these children require an atmosphere that overflows with peace, serenity, benevolence, and structure. I developed the habit of avoiding jerky movements myself, of speaking softly, of smiling often, of making my requirements for each child absolutely clear so that he always knew what was expected and what to expect of himself. I trained myself to follow the same procedure and schedule day after day, letting the children know about changes far in advance, frequently reminding them that the change was coming and that it was an exception.

What an unfortunate burden many, many of our children bear. But is it only misfortune, a chance happening of nature, that imposes this burden? Does society contribute? Can society accommodate new ways of seeing this handicap and seeing itself in the light of this handicap? Can this burden be lessened or removed? Important questions.

The mind of the learning disabled is as ill-equipped to handle the paradoxes as the brain is. The mind introspects and says, "There is something seriously wrong with me. I see that I am different, with a wrong kind of difference. I see myself as practically worthless to myself or anybody else." I have not known many learning-disabled children with positive, stable, predictable self-images. Among those I have known who have presented this image, I'm sure that some have tricked me. Like Fred, whom you met earlier in this book, they created a "face of confidence." Unlike Fred, they showed me this face only.

The learning-disability paradox cannot be a natural state of affairs. Dull people are not usually bright, paralyzed people do not walk, blind people do not normally see. It is difficult for the literate majority to understand how a "normal" segment of the population can be illiterate.

The human mind-brain (even the small brain and smaller mind found in lower creation) is unbelievably subtle. It should be able to see its way through this subtle paradox that unites normality with illiteracy. But it doesn't. I wonder if the mass mind of our culture (which will not countenance paradoxical situations) has put the learning-disabled child in a no-win situation.

15

The Divided Mind-Brain

FIFTY YEARS AGO one half of a brain was removed from a human skull. The art and science of *hemispherectomy* was born.

Long before this, anatomy showed that nature had divided the human brain into two compartments, equal in size, weight, and configuration. This division does not occur throughout the whole brain, only in the cerebrum. I recall studying that the cerebellum is sort of divided by a roll of cells called the vermis (worm, of all names). But the division of the cerebrum is clear cut, no "sort of" about it.

Hemispherectomies began to be performed around the third decade of this century and proliferated to the benefit of brain-tumor patients who preferred to be living bodies with a half brain to corpses with all of it. Neurosurgeons have learned much about brain function from this surgical procedure. They have learned nothing about the mind, however, because they are not sure if the mind lives in half brain, is half brain, or whole brain, or is something universal that uses the brain (whole or half) as long as it lives.

The brain is spherical and its compartments are laterally adjacent to each other, so the compartments were called right and left hemispheres. In actuality, they are not completely separate but joined by cross cables of nerve-filled fibers.

These fibers are called commissures or, collectively, the corpus callosum. The hemispheres communicate with each other through these commissures.

It is surprising that psychologists and educators did not communicate with neurosurgeons during all these years, for surely a divided brain must add something to or subtract something from learning theory. But none of this happened. Until the sixth decade of the twentieth century.

At the California Institute of Technology, Roger W. Sperry, Michael Gazzaniga, Jerre Levy, Colwyn Trevarthen, Robert Nebes, and others (now called the Cal Tech Group) studied a small number of neurosurgical patients whose cerebral hemispheres had been surgically separated (the corpus callosum was cut) to alleviate epileptic seizures involving both hemispheres. Their studies, and others that followed, have pointed new directions for learning theories that were up against mind-brain dead ends. Psychologists and educators continue to find new inspiration in these studies. Even I, a stubborn, pragmatic teacher, ask two questions of each hemisphere. "What can you teach me about learning-disabled children? How will this information help me to help them better?"

I wish I could arrange my answers into neat categories, presenting them in charts, graphs, grids, and computer print-outs. But my answers raise questions, and my questions do not always raise answers. The mind-brain as computer would make this job easier, but the mind-brain is computer plus, plus, plus . . .

The best I can do is to offer a random list of what I have learned, apply this information to learning disability, and attempt a synthesis at the end of the chapter. Bear with me. For the moment, don't try to relate these observations; they are intended to stand alone.

1. The right cerebral hemisphere directs the left side of the body — left leg, left hand, left ear, left eye.

2. The left cerebral hemisphere directs the right side of the body — right leg, right hand, right ear, right eye.

3. The left cerebral hemisphere is usually the language hemisphere, which deals with naming objects, qualities of objects, actions, qualities of actions, and states of being. Since language (and the abstractions and communication of abstractions that language makes possible) is considered the "human element" of our planet, the left hemisphere is called the dominant hemisphere. Patients who have undergone hemispherectomy of the dominant hemisphere usually become what we call "vegetables." The mind is removed, other nonthinking, nonaware functions remain. (I have read that in a very few of these cases the mind has returned from nowhere or somewhere and somehow found the speech to express itself.)

4. Right-handed, right-eyed, right-eared, right-legged people have a left cerebral hemisphere that controls language. In the case of some left-oriented people, and a few with the orientation mixed, the right hemisphere controls language. Some ambidexterous persons use either hemisphere for the language function. All of these are exceptions. They amount to only five percent of the population. (Learning-disabled children comprise perhaps fifteen percent of the school population, so their disability must relate to something *other than* or something *in addition to* lack of left-hemisphere dominance.)

5. In all but a very, very few cases, the language function resides in the left hemisphere only. Most other functions are located in both hemispheres. (This is an unusual arrangement. In case of hemispheric brain injury, almost all functions can be compensated for by the sister hemisphere — except the language function that places us "just a little below the angels." What is the meaning of nature's reckless disregard for a function of such magnitude? Maybe language is such a highly specialized, very

recent addition to our humanness that human neurology hasn't completely assimilated it yet. Maybe language is not all that makes us human, or even the most important thing.)

6. When we are born, the neurological structure necessary for language exists in the right hemisphere as well as in the left. In a child, a major lesion of the left hemisphere produces a transfer of the language function to the right hemisphere. The older the child the less the chance of this happening. After age eight it rarely happens. After age ten it almost never happens. In fact, the area in the temporal lobe of the right hemisphere corresponding to the language area of the left hemisphere appears to have no function at all in adolescents and adults. (The learning-disabled child has great difficulty with either visual language or oral-aural language or both. This indicates a dysfunctioning of the dominant left hemisphere. Early detection and training would appear to be very wise. This is a time during which the right hemisphere might be capable of "picking up the slack.")*

---

*Early detection of learning disability and early training of learning-disabled children have always been difficult areas to research and implement because school failure has been the primary symptom of this disability, and remediation of school failure the principal treatment. The preschool child does not possess the cognitive, perceptual, motor, or language maturity necessary to assess his academic future accurately. Delayed language development is probably the most accurate predictor. When high risk of failure is predicted, no sure way exists, to my knowledge, to turn this risk factor into a success factor before the child's schooling begins. If you are interested in information on current efforts with the three- to five-year-old group, you might contact:

Learning Disability Program
Bureau of Education for the Handicapped
U.S. Office of Education
Washington, DC 20202

The Association for Children with Learning Disabilities
4156 Library Road
Pittsburgh, PA 15234

7. The corpus callosum is not developed until age two. (The foundations of language are laid during the first two years of life. During this period the child develops "object constancy." He learns to perceive differences among objects, then perceives that objects with their particular differences remain the same. He learns to symbolize or create impressions in his mind-brain of objects no longer present to his senses. This symbolization is concrete [actually visualization], but it forms the functional pattern for abstract symbolizing. It is during this period that the child begins to imitate the sound symbols used by adults. Then he goes beyond sound imitation. Using these sounds, he begins to name objects. During the first two years of life, the child also develops an internalized form of sensory motor action, which, combined with body knowing and awareness, enables him to plan movement. This lays the foundation for future concept formation, which is nothing more than planning relationships among semantic elements. All of this foundation building happens without the intervention of the corpus callosum. No learning is passing from hemisphere to hemisphere. Each hemisphere is building the foundation of language — a foundation that will be abandoned in the right hemisphere like a bankrupt building project.)

8. Medical research has indicated for some years now that brain functions can be shaped and reshaped by environ-

The Foundation for Children with Learning Disabilities
L.D. Box 2929, Grand Central Station
New York, NY 10163

Child
15749 N.E. Fourth Street
Bellevue, WA 98008

Academic Therapy Publications
20 Commercial Boulevard
Novato, CA 94947

ment. Surrounding cortical areas can take up functions once assigned to a dysfunctioning area. Sometimes, a functioning area in one hemisphere will substitute for a corresponding area that is dysfunctioning in the opposite hemisphere. At times this transfer of function just happens. Nature has "built in" the back-up mechanism. At other times, transfer is triggered and stimulated by external therapy or training. (Visual and aural-oral language dysfunctions do not seem to transfer naturally, but require triggering or training. For this reason, it would seem to be a mistake to wait for a child to "outgrow" his learning disability, letting nature take its course. There is another good reason why we should avoid this wait-and-see game. The older the brain gets the more set in its ways it becomes. Mind follows brain here. Just as the brain gets used to dysfunction, so the mind gets used to failure. I am hard put to recall an adolescent who just "grew out of" a childhood or preadolescent learning disability. Most that I recall who reached adolescence without help grew into the disability more deeply, both academically and emotionally. Since none of us is sure how, where, or why the brain develops learning disability, we should concentrate great energy on creating, refining, and implementing techniques that stimulate symbol-semantic activity in the brain. Proof that we are using a correct technique is simple. It is not necessary to examine brain patterns. The true test is simply to observe the child. Is he reading, writing, spelling, and speaking better?)

9. Both hemispheres receive language, but only the left hemisphere uses it. I have read accounts of stroke patients with left-hemisphere damage who could not speak, read, or write. Yet these patients could understand language; they were able to follow both oral and picture language. Presurgical procedures that sedate one hemi-

sphere and then the other have also generated empirical evidence that the left hemisphere is the locus of receptive and expressive language. The right hemisphere is receptive only. And reluctantly. The Cal Tech experiments indicate that, except in cases of trauma, the left hemisphere does all the receiving and all the expressing. Yet, in cases of extreme trauma (like left hemispherectomy), the adult mind has, on rare occasions, found its way over to the right hemisphere and forced it to "speak." (It seems that every time man postulates a rule concerning the functioning of his mind-brain-body [a rule based on frequent, solid evidence], nature finds a few exceptions to it. The language foundation built in the right hemisphere during the first two years of life is truly abandoned in maturity. Except . . .)

10. Under conditions stated in number nine, above, it has been discovered that while the left hemisphere prefers to deal in semantics, the right hemisphere is comfortable with melody. When the right hemisphere only is active (as in the sedation procedure) the person cannot talk but can sing. When only the left hemisphere is active, the person can talk but cannot sing. Mind you, the right hemisphere's singing is not usually semantic. Mostly, it is merely a rhythmic repetition of words or sentences, but it can be a mindful duplication of a song once learned and now remembered. (I'm not sure, but I wouldn't be surprised if the right hemisphere were accompanied by some foot tapping and finger accompaniment when singing. Melody generally involves as much of the body as it can. The melody I described earlier seems to engage the left hemisphere as well. It generates a better appreciation of word meanings.)

11. EEG machines can measure which cerebral hemisphere is more active at any given time. While both hemispheres are continually active, a greater level of activity is gen-

erally registered in one hemisphere. This greater level of activity switches from one hemisphere to the other approximately once every minute. Underlying this major transfer of activity, there must be continuous lower level communication between hemispheres so that the right hand knows what the left hand is doing — and the right eye, ear, and leg, also. The corpus callosum is a busy bridge. (This minute-by-minute transfer of activity apparently occurs whether the person is involved in right or left or bihemispheric activity. It is difficult to determine which hemisphere is more engaged when the head is hooked to an EEG machine. Nerve impulses go trucking across the corpus callosum, full or empty, according to a set time schedule. This indicates a perpetual melody of neural movement. The brain-body is full of such melodies. Even two heart cells, separated from each other but still living, can be observed under the microscope pulsing to the same rhythm without any function to perform beyond the pulsing. I am convinced that the natural, functional melody of brain-body is the learning-disabled person's greatest ally in the struggle to master disability.)

12. When you ask a person a question, he must grapple with language inside his head in order to come up with an answer. Therapists use a test to determine which hemisphere a person uses for language. They ask a question and observe the person's eyes. If they move to the right while the person thinks of an answer, he is using his left hemisphere; to the left and he is using his right hemisphere. (In the act of reading the eyes move to the right, for writing too. The left hemisphere apparently controls both processes.)

13. Cal Tech research results indicate that the left hemisphere is analytical (good at breaking down) and the right hemisphere is synthetic (good at pulling together).

The left hemisphere is linear and sequential while the right hemisphere is holistic. (The act of reading is linear. It breaks meaning and logic into segments that occur sequentially. This act must be accomplished by the left hemisphere. It cannot be handled by the right hemisphere, whose function is holistic.)

14. A growing mountain of research into hemispheric functions has uncovered sufficient data and patterns of data to make researchers feel secure in attributing specialized functions to the opposite hemispheres. It is not surprising that these functions often pattern into opposites — the Yin and Yang of Western research. Here follows a listing of those functions that I am aware of:

    a. There is overlapping.
    b. The left hemisphere is analytic; the right is synthetic.
    c. The left gives meaning to a context only in terms of its parts. The right gives meaning to parts only within a context.
    d. The left is verbal as well as analytical; the right is spatial and constructive.
    e. The left deals with verbal abstractions; the right with concrete visual images.
    f. The left attends to and gives meaning to words; the right attends to and gives meaning to facial expression and verbal overtone.
    g. The left produces speech; the right produces song.
    h. The left enjoys logic no matter how grating; the right enjoys melody no matter how illogical.
    i. The left thinks neatly and vertically, moving toward logical conclusions; the right thinks sloppily and laterally. Depending on intuition, it is surprisingly, sometimes crazily, creative.
    j. The left works in a space-time continuum; the right is unaware of time unless forced to deal with it, as in cases of left-brain dysfunction.

k. The left sees cause and effect; the right sees effect and doesn't concern itself with cause.

l. The left is digital; it lines up concepts in logical order, like numbers. The right is analogical. It sees likenesses and relationships. It is the seat of the metaphor.

m. The left takes percepts from the body senses and elevates them to concepts abstracted from "body knowing." The right starts its concepts in the body and finishes them there. Its concepts are the product of physical experience.

n. The left is symbolic, using symbols to represent meaning even when these symbols have no concrete relationship to the meaning. The right is concrete, relating to things as they really are.

o. The left is semantic, assigning meaning to symbols and symbols to meaning. The right is sensuous, attracted to things it can use the body to touch, see, smell, hear, taste, or feel.

p. The left is individual; it creates individual mind. The right is universal; it shares in universal mind, relating directly to creation without self-awareness.

q. The left relates to literate, abstract culture; it is the seat of communication among beings. The right is communal. It relates to universal being; it is the seat of "just being."

In terms of this list, I would be inclined to conclude that learning-disabled children are right-hemisphere children. These children are concrete thinkers. They prefer to manipulate and put together concrete objects rather than to use and relate words. They enjoy constructive drawing as long as their efforts aren't named. They will, however, tolerate naming, sometimes encourage it, if the name identifies objects they have encountered and experienced. They can form vivid visual images of objects, actions, and states that they have experienced deeply enough to link to "body knowing" — objects they have seen, heard, felt, manipulated, taken apart, assembled, rubbed, stretched, caressed, internalized.

These children cannot visualize symbols. How do you "body know" something like that? They also form vivid auditory images of things that they have internalized. They realize that the sound goes with the sight and feel. They cannot, however, auditorialize "ăh" or "ĕh" or "ĭh." What real thing makes sounds like that except adult people like teachers and teaching parents? And these aren't their real sounds.

Learning-disabled children are very adept at perceiving the overtones and hidden meanings of facial expressions and body gestures. (God help the unsure, anxiety-ridden, confused parent and teacher. Better for them to have the expression of a mummy or a sphinx.)

These children love humming and foot tapping and pencil tapping and any kind of rhythm. Many sing very well and dance well as long as the dance doesn't have prescribed steps. Break dancing is *the* dance of the learning disabled. I have seen them do it marvelously.

Learning-disabled children are very creative when they can deal with concrete objects and situations. (Not usually with words.) They are especially creative in the surprising, crazy meaning of creativity. When I see a stalking praying mantis or a feeding frog or a hiding, goggling crab, I imagine that these children understand the bizarre nature of our Creator better than anybody. I remember a twelve-year-old learning-disabled youngster who rigged his boat with foot pedals, oars, a sail, and a rump-controlled rudder. The boat, in or out of operation, looked as bizarre as any praying mantis, frog, or crab. It didn't work as well.

Children who are learning disabled usually live in a space-time vacuum, roving from immediate experience to immediate experience until or unless they become bored. Then they become acutely aware of space and time. "Get away from me. Give me room. What time is it? When's lunch?"

Learning-disabled children do not like to be individual. They prefer to share a natural commonality that most others do not care to share with them. Insects eat each other's eggs, larvae, and each other. Mammals eat each other. Humans eat other mammals. Nobody cares. Learning-disabled children eat each other's lunch (sometimes borrowing a few bites before lunch) and nobody cares, until somebody points it out to a supervising adult. Then all hell breaks loose.

Learning-disabled children do not acculturate easily. They move with nature and immediate inclinations. They are the embarrassment of parents who wonder if others wonder about their upbringing skills and of teachers who worry about their teaching skills.

It is so very tempting to label these children "right-brained" (and "right-minded"). It excuses personal, parental, and teacher guilt just as the "learning-disabled" label has done. It rings with a nostalgia for primitive innocence. There is also a muffled but perceptible undertone: "It's all right to be stupid, dummy. Because you're so sweet and funny."

I am captivated by the "right-brain" concept of learning disability. I want to adopt it as my own. But it doesn't provide enough answers. It doesn't really fit all the problems of these children — only a part of them. For example: The right-brained person is analogical; the learning-disabled child is not. He does not care to compare. Ordinarily, he does not use or appreciate metaphors, especially verbal metaphors.

There are a few exceptions I have known, but these exceptions only add more complexity to our study of humanness. The right-brained person is spatial-visual. He can perceive, duplicate, and remember lines and designs as long as you don't ask him to explain their meaning. Letters, numbers, even words are simple designs. Yet he is hard put to perceive, duplicate, or remember them, even when they are presented bereft of meaning. Is this because his mind-brain sorts out a residue of semantics in the task? Or because he is genetically programmed to snoop out and avoid semantics? I don't know. But I feel that a true, strong, right-brained person should be able to handle the simple design of letters and numbers, regardless.

The right-brained person perceives a gestalt. His perception is global, holistic. But most learning-disabled children cannot remember whole words. My major successes with this kind of child have been analytical. Concentrate on the parts. Remember the whole.

The right-brained person is rhythmic in both the oral-aural and the movement modes of expression. Why, then, does the learning-disabled child read in shreds and write with the finesse of a shredding machine, if he is right brained?

Many learning-disabled children I have known are superb at solving puzzles and winning nonsemantic logic games. (They are often crackerjacks at chess and checkers.) Recently I have discovered that they pick up basic computer programming with surprising adeptness. Admittedly, these tasks are visual-spatial but they are equally logic oriented — a left-brain task.

Most learning-disabled children are better oriented to clockwise movement than to counterclockwise. Primary youngsters most often draw clockwise circles. Draw them a counterclockwise circle, have them draw many such circles and they unconsciously revert to clockwise a short way into the exercise. The most frequent reversals made by learning-disabled children are clockwise reversals for counterclockwise letters. Note the direction of the lateral, curved lines in these letters:

b for d

ↄ for c

ꟻ for f

ꓒ for h

Ꞵ for n

ᘔ for s

But counterclockwise should be a right-hemisphere direction. When our eyes shift left or we use our left ear or move our hand left, we engage the right hemisphere. The learning-disabled child uses eye, ear (he thinks the letter name), and hand when he writes, but his mind-brain prefers to go clockwise. Puzzling, if he is "right brained." It becomes even more puzzling when left-handed learning-disabled children and those with mixed dominance or no apparent dominance at all prefer clockwise — and most of the time they do.

The right-brained person can image and visualize. Why can't the learning-disabled child visualize a letter or number, much less a series of them? The more vivid I make the symbol (using oral expostulations and visual embellishments), the less he remembers it, especially in the long term. But he sometimes remembers the expostulations and embellishments. Why? What happens to letters and numbers in the right or left brain of the learning-disabled child? Back we go again to the semantic connection. Even the "right-brain" theory of learning disability, neat and satisfying as it is, fails when we come to the making of symbols.

It's time to synthesize. It would seem to me that both cerebral hemispheres become involved in different aspects of visual, written, and oral-aural language; that the right hemisphere has some equipment necessary for language as well as the left; that the left is oriented to semantic abstractions and the right to concrete experiential sensations. The right hemisphere apparently is better equipped to handle the spatial, configural, whole-word, whole-sound aspects of language. But it is not oriented to semantics; this seems to have become an atrophied function on the right side.

The right hemisphere sends its package full of the spatial, constructive, gestalt aspects of language to the left hemisphere (there is continuous communion between the two). This package is ordinarily welcomed by a semantic-oriented left hemisphere and language is generated. In the case of the learning-disabled child, however, the left hemisphere is not much more comfortable with semantics than the right; so the package of right-brain elements stays, for the most part, unopened, not processed into symbols, neither semantic for the left nor concrete for the right. Having no meaning for mind to consider or contemplate, these symbols are "washed out" by the mind-brain, and forgotten.

I am postulating that the learning-disabled child is semantically disabled. For some of these children only visual symbols wash out; for some aural symbols wash out; for others all symbols wash out. Symbols have no reason for existing without meaning attached to them. The learning-disabled person can spend a lifetime shuffling symbols in search of meaning.

Perhaps the learning-disabled child is right-brain oriented by necessity, rather than by choice. Because of his semantic difficulty he is insulated at an early age from much of the acculturation of a literate society. He cannot readily make his ideas converge with what the culture values, nor can he readily communicate a growing acculturation to others, for he deals with images and concrete experiences more than with ideas. His inner world is a duplication of his outer world; he is, so to speak, a tissue of sense impressions. Because words do not stuff his hemispheres, he does not constantly juggle them and relate them inside his head. For this reason, he is not very good at using them externally.

I feel that external training (environmental pressure, intensely but judiciously applied) can breathe life and activity into the learning-disabled child's semantic apparatus. (Whatever it is and wherever it is.) This training must stimulate both cerebral hemispheres for a number of reasons. Both hemispheres are in continuous two-way communication; both possess the foundation and potential for symbolic-semantic language; each relegates to the other side the tasks that it would prefer to avoid (and we don't want any tasks left out); both understand language and therefore understand the scope of the task. If the paradoxes of language learning reside in both hemispheres and in their relationships to each other, then these paradoxes can be resolved only by engaging both hemispheres.

Different training approaches have been suggested by concerned researchers and educators. One approach recommends blocking right-hemispheric activity so that it doesn't interfere with left-hemispheric learning. Another recommends engaging the right hemisphere in music so that it is too occupied to interfere. Another suggests retraining the child to left-hemisphere orientation through various cognitive and/or perceptual motor exercises. Another recommends that both hemispheres be engaged in training. I agree with this last approach. Let me add some stipulations:

> The training should be done early, before the right hemisphere forgets that it has a language function.
> The training should be done intensely, so that neither hemisphere has time to go back to its old, separate ways.
> The training should not attempt to restructure the right hemisphere into a left hemisphere on the right side. The use of right-brain functions, in my experience, seems to catalyze the dormant semantic elements of right brain to work in harmony with the active semantic elements of the left.
> One final stipulation. In fact, let's make this stipulation a plea: Don't try to extinguish the right-brain personality of learning-disabled children. They are not deviant. They

are the way they are supposed to be, and the way they enjoy being.

Albert Einstein struggled through his early years in school, then dropped out because he hated it so much. Later, he went back.

Thomas Edison was a school dropout.

Woodrow Wilson admitted that he had many problems in school.

Leonardo da Vinci wrote backward.

Socrates preferred listening and speaking to reading and writing.

What a shame for us, had society changed the personalities of these people, while still young, in "their own best interest."

Much of the information concerning hemispheric functions that I use in observations 1 to 14 was gained from the following sources:

Tony Buzan, *Use Both Sides of Your Brain* (New York: E.P. Dutton, 1976).

Marilyn Ferguson, *The Brain Revolution* (New York: Taplinger, 1973).

Michael S. Gazzaniga, *The Bisected Brain* (New York: Appleton-Century-Crofts, 1970).

Julian Jaynes, *The Origin of Consciousness in the Breakdown of the Bicameral Mind* (Boston: Houghton Mifflin, 1976).

Part Three

Redefining the Learning-Disabled Child

16

A New Definition

THERE ARE LEARNING-DISABLED CHILDREN and there are learning-disabled children. In chapter 4, I defined *learning disability* for the purposes of this book as a disability occurring among people of normal intelligence causing moderate to severe deficits in one, some, or all of the following areas:

reading	attention
spelling	concentration
writing	memory
arithmetic	self-control
spoken language	organization

Let me add a little to this now so that I can make the parameters of my new definition as clear as possible. It is generally accepted that inability to learn is neurologically and/or psychologically caused. Neurological evidence for learning disability is usually referred to as hard or soft. "Hard evidence" is internal evidence: It is central-nervous-system damage or dysfunction that is specifically or approximately located, that is labeled in medical rather than educational terms, and that is treated primarily by medical means. "Soft evidence" is external evidence. In this case, internal dysfunction is inferred from external behaviors such as deficits in the areas listed above. The definition I develop in this chapter should be applied to "soft" learning disability.

Psychological evidence for learning disability may also be referred to as hard or soft, though I have never heard these terms used in a psychological context. The behavior of the person who has withdrawn from the reality he must confront daily (whether concrete or semantic), who is able to deal only with self-created reality, who shows symptoms that readily classify his behavior by psychological label, is "hard." The behavior of the person who is angry, flighty, or uncaring in his dealings with reality, who causes discomfort to others and himself, is "soft." My definition refers to "softly" disturbed children.

Surely there is some crossover between hard neurological/psychological problems and soft educational/behavioral ones. A person may have eye problems with some neurological base, such as amblyopia (lazy eye) or other ocular movement problems; he may have a biochemical problem, such as hypoglycemia. He may have severe coordination problems, even paralysis of some neuromuscular functions. He may be epileptic. If he is generally alert, curious, bright in outlook, average in intelligence (based on tests like the Stanford-Binet, the Wechsler Intelligence Scale for Children [WISC], or the Wechsler Adult Intelligence Scale [WAIS]), and is failing in school, he fits my description of learning disabled.

A child may have a history of psychological and behavioral problems. If he "balances out" (becomes nice when he is apart from such "restrictive environments" as school and home with their learning and organizational demands), if he relates to various concrete tasks in an active and constructive way, if he is average or bright in intelligence, but failing in school, he fits my definition of learning disabled.

Some children may fit many of the above categories yet do well in school; some do not. The difference cannot be the category. It must be the learning disability.

It may seem that I am limiting the scope of learning disability and the number of learning-disabled children. In fact, I
am not. Also in chapter 4, I wrote that learning-disabled children comprise ten percent to twenty-five percent of the childhood population. I stand by this. The percentages go higher if
"hard evidence" children are included. Generally speaking,
my definition fits the educationally accepted norms for learning disability, though many learning-disabled children fitting
this definition are not served in any special way in our
schools. Budgets must be balanced and the number of these
children is so overwhelming that only the worst cases can be
given recognition and special help. (They are usually mixed
with mildly disabled "hard evidence" children.) I suspect that
there is a philosophical reason also. Most of us feel that those
who are almost normal should be normal without any
almost.

Have you ever thought how we are inclined to condemn
ourselves and our most respected professions with the as-
sumptions we make? We declare that one out of four children
has some degree of learning disability. Then we blame the
cause of this learning disability on prenatal, perinatal, or
postnatal insult. Prenatal insult implies that a pregnant
mother was not very careful. Postnatal implies that a new
mother was careless or ignorant. Perinatal implies that a doctor was careless. (Prenatal and postnatal involve a doctor too,
for he advises the pregnant mother on self-care and checks
regularly on the health of the child.) Whatever the cause,
smoking, lifting, anoxia at birth, high fever, undetected ear
infections, and on and on, we are implying that the parents
and doctors of this very advanced and literate society are to
blame for the dysfunctioning of up to twenty-five percent of
our children. Hard to accept. I cannot accept it. I have a learning-disabled child and refuse to blame my wife, myself, or
any doctor.

Genetics sits better with me. Humans are born with predis-
positions for all kinds of things, even a predisposition for sa-

voring an object rather than its name. You know, as well as I, that we all start out this way. Object is everything. Bite it, gum it, smell it, see and touch it, drop it, grab it, shake it, pinch it, hear it, swallow it, digest it, excrete it, until somebody names it over and over and we imitate their naming. Most of us swing over to the "naming game" with delight. Some of us trudge over grudgingly, still preferring the real thing to the name. In an infant, it is unlikely that this happens by psychological choice. Genetic inclination is more likely. I mentioned earlier that new evidence indicates that some cell dysplasia in the left cerebral hemisphere might possibly (still a very long shot) cause this inclination. Can't dysplasia be inherited?

The learning-disabled child is a modern paradox! He would have been a long-standing — even ancient — paradox, had previous generations upon generations expected everybody to be efficiently literate in a literate society. We moderns say that this child has a sensory problem; yet he lives more than any of the rest of us in his senses. We say that he has a reality-adjustment problem; yet he adjusts to the real sensory world, actually thrives in it (sometimes wallows in it) better than most of the rest of us. We say that he is "spaced out," doesn't know what is going on in the world of "real people." Yet, as an infant he was probably among the first in the neighborhood to recognize faces. As a child he is the best at reading them. He will read "weak, uncaring, just-a-job-or-obligation, sarcastic, burned-out, despairing" faces, and if these are the faces forcing him into unpleasant, confounding, self-image killing, semantic situations, he will gain the advantage with the shrewdness of the fox and the web-making of the spider. (Beware parent and teacher. I speak as both.) He will also read "concerned, trying, I-won't-give-up, I-love-and-respect-you-as-you-are" faces and respond to instruction. (But beware here, also, parent and teacher. If you don't effectively commit yourself and your time to helping him overcome his disability he'll figure that he misread your face just as he misreads your words.)

The learning-disabled child has always been identified by negatives, even by all of us who have tried and tried and tried to understand him, cope with him, and live with him at school and at home. We have called him *in*attentive, *un*comprehending, *im*mature, *dis*organized, *un*grateful, *dis*obedient, *un*remembering, *dis*inhibited, *un*careful, *un*caring, *dys*lexic, *dys*graphic, *dys*calculic, *un*cooperative, *un*predictable, and *un*happy. Let's close our eyes for a moment to our accustomed world of learning disability and the perceptual sets of that world. Let the *in*'s, *un*'s, *dis*'s, *im*'s, and *dys*'s of that world float free of us. We'll be observers. We'll sit back comfortably. We'll forget all labels, all etiologies, all diagnoses, all interventions. Then we'll open our eyes to a new world of *special learning ability*. Let's imagine that we can see the inner and outer workings of the mind-brain. We observe a child (let's call him our child) who is shamefully uninterested in words but purely devoted to objects named by those words. A child bored to silliness by abstractions, but a wholehearted observer of the real things that foster abstractions. Our child uses words, often overuses them, not to analyze or generalize, but to sing, shout, and repeat the praises of the real creatures that are forever appearing to him and the real events that are forever happening. Other children are saying "because," "although," "when," and "therefore." He is saying "alleluia!" Other children retreat inside themselves to think as school and home taught them. He retreats outside himself to experience in spite of what he has been taught.

Our child wanders around whatever part of creation he happens to exist in (classroom and home parts included) without the steady burden of introspection. He is comfortable with creation and creatures because he is not divided from them by constant, nagging self-consciousness. Time does not concern him because he does not measure what he does in segments. Every event is a whole event. The next one always comes, but is not anticipated.

Our child is inclined to neglect his mental dictionary because "in head" movies are more easily available to him. Why read the book when you can see the picture? Especially when the picture is a documentary of a real event and the book a once-, twice-, three-times-removed listing of suppositions about the event.

Our child's mind-brain-body is inclined toward seeing, hearing, touching, smelling, biting, feeling internally whatever he encounters. He stores visual, auditory, and kinesthetic impressions of these encounters that enrich and encourage further encounters. He compares these encounters as any active mind-brain will do. He creates concrete analogies (called metaphors in semantic terms) that will generate further analogies that can suggest new concrete solutions to old concrete problems that can't be solved by words.

Our child can read the real face of reality but cannot read the symbols we have created to represent and analyze that reality. He would seem to connect with the flow of creative evolution that we have jumped out of for the sake of our higher semantics.

Our child apparently retained some of the genes we left behind when we took our giant step forward into the mental processes that substitute names for real things and the introspection that came with naming ourselves. Perhaps he is a mind-brain-body missing link, tying us to the flow of creation as we shoot for the stars. Or as we build our towers of Babel, lest we forget, lest we forget . . .

Let's go back to our known world of learning disability. There is no doubt that our child in this world can be sloppy, uncomprehending, and truculent. We would probably act likewise in his world. He lives in his senses more than his brain, his brain more than his mind. We are more mind than brain, more brain than senses. Neither of us has the whole picture. But I'll bet that, left alone, our child would enjoy his living more than most of us.

The new definition: Learning disability is a normal psycho-physiological condition that inclines the mind-brain-body to favor the experiences and imagings of concrete reality over symbolic/semantic representations of that reality.

17

A Fresh Approach at School

IN OUR SOCIETY and most societies, a school's primary function is to initiate children into the culture of its society. With very few exceptions, the bedrock of this culture is semantic. Children must become facile with words before they are trusted to understand the norms and values of their culture. They must deal efficiently with every form of verbal communication before they are declared ready to take their place in society.

If the child falters or fails in this requirement, parents are ashamed of the school; the school is ashamed of the parents; society is ashamed of both parents and school; everybody is ashamed of the child. (Unless his handicap is so apparent that nobody expects a high degree of semantic learning. The learning-disabled child is not such a child.)

Because the learning-disabled child (labeled or not) is considered normal or almost normal, he is a cinch to cause shame and blame. The energy he generates at school and at home is laden with an aura of embarrassment; he embarrasses himself and those responsible for his cultural growth. He is the subversive in the camp of culture, for he is not easily acculturated and tends (especially at school) to subvert, by clever example, the cultural growth of other children.

School officials have no choice but to crush his will. To let him remain as he is without effort to change him is to negate educational/cultural philosophies, purposes, and practices. For this reason, educators must start with the premise that the learning-disabled child is wrong, a bad apple. Most educators do not feel that he is intentionally bad, at least when he is a young child. They recognize that their very efforts to cultivate him cause much of the badness, but cultural values and demands leave them no choice but to proceed with the process. Occasionally they are successful; more often they are not. The learning-disabled child, in time, becomes less *impulsive* in his attempts to avoid the process and more *compulsive* in his attempts to undermine it. After he leaves school (sometimes before), he will choose, more often than we like to think, to undermine culture at large. The prison and delinquency studies I mentioned earlier bear this out. Most learning-disabled people, of course, do not choose this. They choose to endure "the slings and arrows of outrageous fortune." Some, in spite of everything, become successful. Human nature is very resilient.

Parent and teacher checklists used to help diagnose the problem of learning disability are evidence that learning disability is regarded as a negative influence, no good for the afflicted child or anyone else. Here is a sampling of qualities or behaviors culled from a cross section of these lists, presented in no particular order:

immature	quarrels
lazy	fights
sloppy	cries
overactive	wets the bed
destructive	aggressive
doesn't complete	withdrawn
assignments	poor memory
disorganized	doesn't pay attention

is too loud	uses vulgar language
impulsive	has developed facial tics
uninhibited	irresponsible
creates embarrassing	angry
situations	frustrated
disobedient	irrational fears
uncooperative	sneaky
below grade level in some	careless
or all subjects	uncaring
clumsy	unhappy
uncoordinated	accident prone
rude	hard to like

What a monster this child is! Is he a bad seed? Or has culture made him this way? Do we so worship our cultural values that we will unwittingly and unwillingly make a monster of a child? Important questions; value questions that exceed the demands of any culture — questions of the human spirit.

In answer, I will declare forthrightly that I have not been dealing for more than twenty-seven years with bad seeds. Different seeds, yes, but not bad. I am also convinced that we have valued our cultural expectancies and acceptance more than we have valued some of our children. Not only parents and educators bear responsibility. Every one of us who says "Hammer culture into the child who dares to refuse it!" shares some responsibility for the sufferings and distortions of these children. Thousands of times I have heard learning-disabled children say, "Why don't you, they, just leave me alone?"

Leaving alone, of course, is not the answer. But I can suggest a way to invite these children back into a society that has declared them unfit. Why don't we search out their positive qualities? We don't have to search far. Why don't we begin our diagnoses with positive checklists? Here is one presented in no particular order:

loves animals
caring of younger children
caring of handicapped
works well with hands
explores the mechanism
   (workings) of any
   concrete object
creative
affectionate
honest to the point of being
   blunt
curious
loves life right here in the
   present
optimistic
courageous
humorous
loves to sing
loves to move
draws well
exuberant
cheerful
caring
close to nature
loves himself
loves water
loves air, wind, breezes,
   weather
loves wood
loves insects
loves reptiles

loves amphibians
loves stones
loves dirt
loves people
loves to see
loves to hear
loves to smell
loves to touch
loves to talk
loves to play
loves to smile
loves to laugh
is interesting
is interested
is original
is perceptive
wants to contribute
wants to share

Some positive negatives:

unselfish
nonjudgmental
not rigid
doesn't have to be right
unsarcastic
not argumentative
doesn't hold grudges
not boring
not bored
not guilt-ridden

Whenever I have lifted the semantic/cultural burden from learning-disabled children for hours or for days they have put on my positive list like a well-fitting suit, eagerly and immediately. Whenever I have turned the semantic screws, they have put on the worst of their culture, like strait-jacketed inmates. What an instant metamorphosis in both directions! What a dilemma for parent and teacher! Take off cultural pressure and he is nice. Apply it and he is a monster. Is there any escape? I think so.

The learning-disabled child wants to be like "everybody else." He will undergo much duress to master the "cultural set" expected of him if he feels that he has a chance to master it. This chance was the one thread (a thread that turned into a cable) that gave me support as a child through years of embarrassment, worry, fear, and very hard work. And through the many successes and failures in my teaching career, I have never lost my conviction that learning disability can be conquered. I have permeated my efforts with a "we will overcome" feeling. Some years ago a student of mine created a class anthem that we sang (and that I still sing with learning-disabled children on occasion) with gusto and conviction.

> *This handicap*
> *Is a bum rap,*
> *I won't put up with it anymore!*
> *If you think my mind's slow*
> *Or my talents low,*
> *Sir, I'll show you to the door.*

(I changed this line; the original was, "Sir, I'll knock you to the floor.")

> *We want the world to know*
> *We got a lot to give.*
> *Sir, if you think this is bull*
> *It's your brain that's the sieve.*

So *Step One*, which will enable us concerned educators, parents, and citizens to break through our dilemma, is to hold out to our learning-disabled children the hope, the probability, that they can become as semantic as culture demands.

Step Two I will reserve for Part Four of this book. It is essential that we face this hopeful child with a procedure that works. I feel that I have found one such procedure, and there are others. These must be the procedures that are used and used intensively. A little bit of this procedure and a little bit of that, applied cautiously ("Don't upset the child"; "Don't expect too much") *will* upset the child and won't help him learn anything. Overcoming learning disability is a whole-hog affair. For the sake of the child, we must go at it with conviction. If we doubt the child or ourselves, or our procedure, we are "whistling Dixie." The learning-disabled child will read us with an insight that belies his inability to read our books. And he will treat us and our attempts just as the wind treats a gardener sowing seeds.

Step Three is essential to the success of steps one and two. We are dealing with an upside-down process or, more precisely, an amalgamated process. Without the catalytic influence of step three, step one becomes a faith-laden jump into an uncertain void. Step two becomes meaningless "head noise" that aggravates rather than alleviates. Step three is so obvious that we almost always overlook it. It is the self-worth builder, the "so what if I fail, I'm still worth something" assurance. It is a cultural life insurance policy for the learning-disabled child. It tells him, "Even if you fail, your self-image will survive." In step three, we provide the child with many opportunities to do what he naturally does best. And we give these activities at least equal billing with semantic activities. They are not to be icing on the cake, but a part of the cake itself. The learning-disabled child will enjoy them as any child enjoys licking icing. But we must be convinced that these activities are more than icing. We should not tell the child that overeager ingesting of these activities will "ruin his semantic supper." Neither should we make this "dessert" a reward for finishing supper. Let me suggest some appropriate activities:

1. Hands-on natural science, with many opportunities for observation, hearing, touching, probing, and microscoping for a closer look. Science with open-ended exploration and without conclusion-making reports.
2. Art without guidelines, giving help only when help is requested.
3. Physics without lab books. Open-ended physics that encourages tinkering, taking apart, putting together. Try-and-try-again physics that doesn't demand "Do it this way" or "It should turn out this way."
4. Field trips without guides, only monitors.
5. Computer play (if the school can afford it) without much instruction until the child asks for instruction.
6. Social studies activities that begin with concrete experiences, encourage concrete analogies, and end with concrete conclusions, whatever they may be.
7. Social activities that involve singing, movement, and interaction without goals and the burden of rules unless the law or individual rights and sensibilities are being violated. This is unlikely since learning-disabled children are quite sensitive to the feelings of others.

I'll stop here, but all of us can, I am sure, think of many other suitable activities.

Would it be possible for the schools, which we have created as paragons of cultural initiation, to use some initiative on behalf of ten, maybe fifteen, percent of our children? Would we allow our schools to restructure a part of themselves for a part of our children? Could we permit them to institute "special-learning" classes instead of "learning-disability" classes? Could the children in these classes be considered an asset to the school rather than a threat? Could they receive hope-filled, intensive, semantic training for part of the day, and be themselves for the rest? They would become the envy of the school, I am sure, for their program would raise nostalgia in the other students (even some teachers) for a part of human-ness left behind when we became more like the angels — and also more like the devils. Could we tolerate this? Are we afraid to give words to a minority who might teach us how to live and enjoy each moment? Who might teach us that we have gone too far, too fast? That life is experiencing, and bringing inside, and experiencing more? And knowing? Starving insects and mammals eat their brood. We may have outgrown this. Yet we let our culture gobble up that segment of our brood that inherits a mind-brain-body preference for direct experience rather than for reading and writing.

We are self-aware beings. If we can't romanticize (fall in love with) our existence, no wonder that we unwittingly create a culture that devours children who point backward rather than forward. We are moderns, often growing in the air without roots, breathing abstractions. But abstractions are not the oxygen of our existence. We are not rarefied enough for this yet. Old elements must mix with our abstract atmosphere and influence it and create new (rooted) possibilities. I believe that learning-disabled children, born and bred every day, connect us with our existential past. We can lift them to our semantic heights. We should. But we should also let them remind us of our connection with real existence.

Can our schools do this for us? Only if we let them.

18

Persevering at Home

IN THE HOME, the learning-disabled child often causes guilt and feels guilt. His parents blame themselves for the way he is, and the child does not rest easy with the "bad me" image that his behavior warrants and his family sometimes fosters. Dad and Mom love him, without doubt, but they cannot let him (or themselves) forget that he is not a chip off the old cultural block. For, after all has been said and done, almost all parents want their offspring to be offshoots of the culture that defines them. It is the lot of the learning-disabled child to be a poor definition or a wrong definition of this culture. It is his lot to cause his parents to doubt their upbringing skills and to worry about the judgment of others upon this incompetence.

Shortly after the birth of a child, parents look for the buds of linguistic competence to sprout so that they can encourage their growth. "Daddy, Mommy, finger, smile, eat." But the new baby is too enthralled with Daddy and Mommy's faces to listen. Too busy using the finger to name it. Too busy smiling or crying in the face of experience to attend to distractions. Too busy tasting to name the act that makes it possible. While the mind-brain of the neighbor's baby is willing and able to set aside a portion of the real world for a word-built world, just as the new baby's older sister or brother did, this new baby's mind-brain is not inclined this way. Sure, an occasional (even frequent) expostulation of surprise or delight is emitted, but no dogged determination to imitate the sounds of Mom and Dad. "Bad you" is the result. "We love you and we're going to try harder to make you talk." But still "bad you." Parents look for their newborn to grow into a toddler. Now that you have rolled over, crept, crawled, it is time to toddly walk, toddly run, toddly lunge, toddly jump, toddly fall. All the things involved in toddling. But the new child does not go through the toddler stages in any sequence. He goes through all stages without sequence. He walks when he should be crawling, creeps when he should be walking, rolls when he should be upright; he is backward and precocious at the same time. He is not developmentally delayed but developmentally scrambled. His parents have not produced a "normal" child but a whirlwind. One that takes things when it shouldn't take them and breaks things when it shouldn't break them. "Bad you" for this.

The new child enters preschool. He is too rough (too exploring?) with things, too rough with other children. Or he is too withdrawn, too contemplative. He is too much work for the teacher and affects (infects?) other children. Send him home. The teacher is tired. The parents are embarrassed. "Bad you" again.

The child enters school. Read, child, read. Write, child, write. Buffer your real world with a semantic world. Name a pencil instead of chewing it, name a bug instead of going and finding it, name a feeling instead of feeling it, name a classmate in place of knowing him. Talk to yourself inside your head instead of listening to the talk of everything outside your head. The child's mind is tired of being bad, so it tries. But the brain remains outdrawn and will not cooperate. The child does not learn to read and write as rapidly as the other children. The teacher is sad or mad. The parents are embarrassed. "Bad you," says the teacher. "Bad you," say the parents. The teacher regrets, but just a little. The parents regret a lot, for they need verification of their life investment and are not getting it. The child is confused a lot. "Where do I go from here?" he asks. "Do I play mind games with the cultural world and live a 'fake life,' do I steel myself and continue trying to 'really make it' in this awful, awesome world of head words, or do I follow my brain outside and continue being bad? Where do I go from here?"

The parents ask the same question. They ask it over and over as their child jumps from one intervention to another as he grows older. Unfortunately, parents cannot afford the luxury of multiple approaches. Culture prescribes a path and all who are respectable follow it and impart it to their offspring. Respectable parents of learning-disabled offspring live an awful dilemma, just as their offspring do. "Love my child or love my culture?" asks the parent. "Love myself or love my parents?" asks the child. What bitter choices! Just *being* should be so simple, so natural, enough for both of them. But culture will not allow this simplicity. Culture-bound as they are, they ask (we ask, I ask) for cultural solutions.

Let me suggest some ways to perceive and handle the learning-disabled child at home that can be fulfilling personally and culturally. Not ultimate solutions, but suitable to us where we find ourselves right now. Anything I suggest on the following pages I have tried with my own learning-disabled child — successfully up to this point, Saturday, March 31, 1984, 2:10 P.M. Things could change for the worse. I don't think they will.

Parents of learning-disabled children should, first and foremost, erase the "bad guy" image from their minds and the child's, whether it be active "bad guy" image or poor little helpless "bad guy" image. This is not difficult to want to do, for in dealing with our child we deal from the heart. It is actually not difficult to do, either. Parents should review the positive checklist from the last chapter, even use it to check off and mull over the good and exciting qualities in their learning-disabled child. They should add to the list as they rediscover the child. Finally, they should find occasion to share the world of their child. It will be exhilarating to live right now, instead of dissolving the moment in a head dialogue between past and future. It will be heady to live in the senses instead of talking inside the head. It will feel serene to enjoy a good startle but not to carry fear; to be curious, but not to worry.

The child will be suspicious at first. The sudden change in behavior will smell fishy. But the parent should persevere. The smell soon evaporates in the clear air that he has created.

Now life is more livable for both child and parent. But the learning-disabled child must still be acculturated. His home may be willing to accept new awareness, but his culture is not. The social selves of the parent and child must swim in the culture or sink. It's the only ocean they have and it will have to do until they and God and all of us evolve a new one.

So we parents must turn somewhere for help. Where else but to psychology? In my opinion, we must be careful, because some psychology is still totally behavior oriented and we can be drawn into a behavior-changing morass. (After all, changing our child's behavior is our intent.) I am leery of a strictly behavioral approach. Its premise scares me because it says that mind does not exist. It recognizes only brain, receiving and being shaped by controlling stimuli. There is much truth to this premise. Consider how we are shaped by our culture in spite of the cries of our children. But my bias is a result of my personal philosophy. I keep thinking of minds that persuaded brains to take giant leaps in the face of cultural conditioning. (Many of these minds, by the way, have been "learning-disabled" minds persuading "learning-disabled" brains.)

But back to the issue at hand. It's time for practical suggestions to parents of learning-disabled children. My advice is fourfold. It includes one "Thou shalt not" and three "Thou shalts."

1. Thou shalt not reward or withhold attention from thy child on the basis of his annoying behaviors. What I am saying is directly contrary to psychological practice in some circles of influence. I am saying that behavior-modification programs do not ordinarily work well with SLD children. There are several reasons for this:

   a. The child himself cannot internalize control over his behavior at the behest of a reward or the withdrawal of your attention. He will no doubt like the reward and dislike losing your attention. He will make great tearful, heartfelt promises about reforming and mean them. Yet five minutes later he'll be into it with his sister again or dropping his clothes all over the house.

   b. Any effective behavior-modification program must be enforced rigorously. You must be in a position to observe every target behavior and be disposed to take appropriate action in every instance. You won't be able to. Your child will wear you down.

   c. If there are siblings in the family, they won't let you implement an effective behavior-modification program either. They will become upset at the special treatment given to "Mama's pet" just because he's so freaky. Should you try to include them in the program too, either they'll rebel because they're not freaky or they'll start acting freaky so you'll be more aware of their good behavior and quicker with the reward. (If you're good all the time, you're taken for granted.)

   d. If you persist in trying to "modify" your learning-disabled child's behavior, he will interpret *your* behavior as manipulation. (In a sense it is, even though your motive is noble.) He can very easily learn manipulation as a lifestyle. Some of the worst little manipulators in my classes (disliked immensely by fellow students, liked only with extreme effort by the teacher) were children who were undergoing behavior modification at home.

2. Thou shalt make thy home life as structured as possible. For some of us this seems almost as difficult as implementing a behavior-modification program. We free spirits like to come and go when we please, eat when we feel like it, spend time with the kids when we're in the mood. Unfortunately, some of this freedom will have to go for a while, but it won't be as difficult as it sounds. In between the structured points of the day you can be as free as you're accustomed to being. Besides, maintaining a schedule is really a whole lot easier than modifying behavior. Structuring home life means arranging for the same events to happen at the same time each day. Breakfast and dinner should be scheduled; so also should be homework time, chore time, TV time, waking time, and bedtime. This does not mean that *you* have to follow this schedule. You follow only the parts that you do with the children; the rest you enforce. This does not mean, either, that you cannot make exceptions to the schedule, like going out to dinner, visiting friends, having friends over, or going out for a day or a weekend. Just be sure not to make every day an exception and make sure that the child knows in advance that an exception is coming — and that it is an exception. Do not try to structure your home only for your learning-disabled child. Do it for all of your children. It is beneficial to the child without learning disability; it is essential to the learning-disabled child. For years, I have structured both my class and my home. All of the many SLD children I have worked with,

including my daughter, have gained from structure and developed a lifestyle, a perception of how the parts of life fit together and progress, that has in turn helped them develop a structured perception of symbols and their sequences.

3. Thou shalt train thy child to do chores according to schedule — not just assign them and hope. If your children (especially the one who is learning disabled) are like mine, you spend a good part of your waking hours and even a larger part of your energy shouting monologues like this: "Pick up those socks; pick up those shoes; don't leave your underpants on the kitchen floor; clean your room and don't shove everything under the bed; take out the trash. Oh! the truck already came; feed the dog; get your dirty hands off the walls; you said you were going to weed around those bushes a month ago; now I can't even see the bushes. Sweep the garage. That's your job. I don't even remember what color the floor is. Why is there peanut butter on the ceiling? All you did was make a sandwich. Stop treating your sister like an animal; when are you going to put away the dishes, and don't break any like last time; when is the last time you made your bed? You probably don't even know where it is with all the junk on top of it." These monologues go on and on. Nobody listens or answers. Spouting them can become an awful drag. The sad thing, you are thinking, is that your SLD child is getting worse at meeting his few simple responsibilities, not better.

I learned something many years ago in the classroom that should be of help to you in this regard. When I started teaching learning-disabled children, I would give an explanation or two, give an assignment on the basis of the explanation, advise everybody to work quietly and raise their hands if they needed help. The only part of my spiel that penetrated was the last. Every hand would be up as soon as the word *help* left my mouth. I felt like calling for help myself. I soon learned that the children would learn only if I helped each one of them through every step of every procedure until they knew the procedure as well as I did. It often became impossible to do this with each child, one at a time, so we would work together at a procedure, I at the board, the students at paper on their desks, step by step, over and over. I would tell them to raise their hands when they were positive they could do it on their own. One by one, they did. Before long I was able to go through it again individually with the one or two who still weren't ready for independence.

How can this experience be of help to the beleaguered parent? If you are one of these, your learning-disabled child will learn to meet his responsibilities *if you go through them with him.* When he gets up in the morning, make the bed with him (not for him). Remind him that this is what he does as soon as he gets up. When he leaves a mess somewhere, clean it up *with him* as soon as you realize that he made it. When it's time to take out the trash, do it *with him* as you alert him to the time. Feed the dog *with him.* Note for him the time the feeding is taking place. When he plays a game with his sister or brother, play along with both of them so that they can perceive how to get along. Whatever responsibilities you wish your learning-disabled child to meet, at whatever time, meet them with him and alert him to the time. (Not necessarily 9:00 A.M. or 7:00 P.M., but "as soon as you get up" or "after supper.")

I can hear you grumbling. I don't blame you. You have your own responsibilities and this sounds like a lot of work. Really it's not. You know as well as I do that you expend more energy trying to force your child to meet responsibilities and doing them for him when he doesn't (which is most of the time) than you do by doing them along with him. "But," you ask, "will I do these chores with him as long as he lives with me?" No, you won't. Eventually, he will put his hand up (so to speak) and say, "Mom (or Dad), I can do this alone at the right time." And he will. Or he may not say anything, but just start to get the job done before you get there. Or sooner or later you may have to say, "Son, can you do this by yourself? Let me know when you can." He'll let you know sooner than you would expect. In a few individual cases, it may be necessary to wean the child from your company one task at a time. If you persist you will win. I won, and most parents who followed this advice have won also. In many cases a special closeness developed between parent and child. What a welcome bonus.

4. Thou shalt be thy child's support and guide during homework sessions — not his teacher. Please do not ever, EVER, become your child's teacher if he has a learning disability. If you do this you threaten and may destroy your parent-child relationship for a while or forever. Remember, injured relations between parent and child that are carried into the child's adolescence sometimes never heal — and adolescence comes very fast. When you teach your SLD child his homework you are approaching him with your parent-love, parent-concern, and parent-power at his weakest point intellectually and emotionally. His unstable self-image has you probably as its only anchor.

"Well," you're probably thinking, "if I don't teach what do I do when my child doesn't know enough to even begin his homework? Tell him to forget it and teach him irresponsibility? Let him fail his class?"

In the arena of learning disability there is one main responsibility — to try to overcome, not to let the child sink in, a sea of semantics. There is one main failure — not to try. All other concerns about responsibility or failure must be subordinated to these.

When your SLD child has a homework assignment, don't

teach it to him, don't even teach him parts of it. Do it with him. I mean this literally. As you do it, he does it. You have one sheet of paper; he has another. In the case of math, you do the problem step by step on your paper and he does it step by step on his paper. Don't say, "Now try one all by yourself." If you do, you're leaving parent behind and becoming teacher. If he tells you that he'd like to do a problem by himself or that he can finish the assignment by himself, let him. If he gets some wrong answer, don't go back and teach him those problems, just keep going on, but slow down your pace.

I am not making a blanket condemnation of parent teaching. I am sure that in some instances parents have done an excellent job doubling as teachers. I am simply expressing my conviction, based on experience, that parents of learning-disabled children are seldom successful when they assume primary responsibility for the education of their learning-disabled child. For they are working too close to the cutting edge of emotion and self-worth.

I recommend this undertaking only in the most dire circumstances and shortly I suggest when it might be considered and how it can be accomplished.

If the assignment is reading, read while he reads. Read slowly, with expression, directly into his ear and he should be able to say each word as he hears it. Don't ask him questions afterward. If you want him to think about what he has read, you think about it out loud. Just let him listen. If he wants to comment on the passage or *ask you* questions, all the better. Listen to his comment; answer his questions. But please don't say, "How can you ask a question like that? We just read . . ."

If the assignment is writing a report or answering questions at the end of a chapter, you write the report or answer the questions and he writes them word by word after you. If he wants you to change something, change it. Think out loud as you are writing these assignments so he can see how you're finding the information and organizing it. Don't question him or have him repeat ideas back to you. If your child has difficulty with handwriting (and he probably does), make your answers as short as you can, even one word. Don't be teacher. Be good old supportive, loving Mom or Dad.

If your child must study for a spelling test, let him give you the test and correct it from his word list. Miss some words on purpose, especially the ones you are sure will cause him the most trouble. In this way, you'll at least be sure that he is examining these words closely as he corrects your paper. Let him know that you're going to miss some words before you take the test. You don't want him to think that he inherited his problem. Take the test again to give him extra practice, missing different words and some of the same ones.

If he wants to take the test, let him. If he misspells some words, simply write the correct spelling after his word while you say the word. Don't say, "If you would only sound it out." Don't become teacher.

I explained the emotional implications of being a parent-teacher earlier. From a purely academic point of view, you will not succeed as teacher. You will confuse your child if your method of instruction is different from his teacher's. You will make him very anxious if he has to answer to you as well as his teacher, and he will be more likely to flub the test or assignment when he feels doubly accountable. How many times have I heard a parent tell me, "Last night I taught him every one of those words; he knew them perfectly. Today he missed twenty out of twenty-five on the spelling test."

To you teachers of SLD children who are reading this, don't become upset with parents who work with their SLD children in this manner. Don't say, "I gave the assignment to James, not his mother." If James went home and couldn't do the assignment on his own, you shouldn't have given it to him in the first place. If you're certain that James can do the assignment and is conning his mother, tell her so that she can stay clear of him during homework time.

These suggestions will help parents to acculturate their learning-disabled children. They usually work when the parent perseveres. Keep in mind that it is easier to persevere when the learning-disabled child is considered a source of information as well as a commodity of reformation. My propensity to learn from the learning disabled has made me a die-hard teacher and parent. Parents, guardians of the home, you have hope in the face of learning disability. But don't only hope. Experience, enjoy, and grow as you acculturate your child; and be sure that your experience absorbs culture, before culture standardizes your experience. If your project turns to a discussion of attitudes or a need for change, it will surely sink.

There is an exception to the foregoing recommendations. It happens, more often than I like to think about, that a learning-disabled child has a single teacher or a group of teachers who do not understand him or his disability. This is bound to happen, of course, when the child struggles in the mainstream. Teachers are not trained to recognize his difficulty or to help him overcome it. But it also happens to learning-disabled children who receive resource help or who have been placed full time in SLD classes. Some teachers, in spite of specialized training, do not understand learning disability, nor do they understand how to approach it. This may be the fault of the teacher or the training, but in either case, the child is getting nowhere. His academics are regressing as well as his behavior. After this has been happening for two months or so (parents shouldn't be impulsive, but neither should they be shy), the parents should, first of all, make their feelings heard, loudly and convincingly, to anybody who has decision-making power in the school their child attends. If this does not get positive results — a change in program, a change in teacher attitude, a change in teacher (and changes aren't always for the better) — they should storm the district offices, time and time again, until a positive change happens. For sure, they will be called names by some secretaries, teachers, and administrators — "the parents who think they have a genius (if they only knew)"; "the parents who think their kid is the only one in the world"; "the parents who have no better way to spend their time"; "the parents who dote on their kid and should let him grow up (into what?)." But if the parents are lucky, they may find somewhere in the administrative offices a tried and true "child advocate" who might find the right placement for their child. "I think, if I pull strings," the advocate says, "I might be able to squeeze him in with Mrs. Hoffman or Mrs. Malavasi, even though their classes are already way overcrowded." As Juan of "Juan's words" would say, "God blast Mrs. Hoffman and Mrs. Malavasi." Of course they have overcrowded classes. The child advocate, knowing and wise, has been sending to them every learning-disabled child he could. Better seventeen with them (add on an aide or two) than one with Mrs. Holsum or Mr. Scruggs. Hoffman and Malavasi understand; they persevere; they judge themselves as readily as they judge students; they get results.

But even very loud and very convincing parents can fail. When this happens, the parents might seek out a private, special school, as second choice, if they can afford it. (These schools range from $5000 to $9000 for daytime help. Residential schools can cost up to $25,000 a year.) You can request that your school district pay this tuition under Public Law 941, which quite simply states that the school district must provide an appropriate education for each special student or must pay for that education elsewhere. It has become increasingly difficult in many states to obtain this financial help. (Five years ago, I had twenty-five students funded under Law 941. Last year, I had one.) School districts are working hard to upgrade learning-disability departments and are understandably reluctant to admit that their programs are inappropriate. You may have to go the "due process" route, which will take much time (important time to the child) and will necessitate engaging a lawyer. You may lose anyway. It is often difficult to prove that a private school has a "more appropriate" program for your child than the public school does. Nobody will know this for sure until the child experiences the private program for a while — and how can this happen if you can't afford it or the district won't pay? In spite of what I say above, it is your right to challenge your school district. The decision is yours.

If you decide to apply to a special private school (hear me, you parents out there), interview the school! Don't let it interview you. Show whatever evidence you have that your child has a learning disability — psychological tests, report cards, teacher comments, your own observations. Listen politely to descriptions of programs, facilities, and qualifications; then go straight to the heart of the matter.

"May I have a student roster with names and phone numbers of other parents who have students here? I would like to know if these parents feel that their children are benefiting from the school."

Don't accept selected names. If the administrator won't let you walk off with a copy of the list, copy names and numbers at random from his master list. Then call the numbers. Open with the statement, "I'm thinking of enrolling my child at your child's school." Then ask three questions:

"Is your child happy there?"

"Is he improving academically?"

"Do you expect him to be able to leave the school soon, if he wants to or if you want him to, and 'make it' in regular school?"

If all of the answers are yes, enroll your child in that school tomorrow. It's worth the money. If you receive a lot of no answers to the first question, the school should be closing soon — for good. Many yeses to the first question and noes to the other two indicate that you might be getting yourself and your child into a "happy farm" environment. Lots of nourishing, but not much growth. You certainly should avoid this.

Yeses to questions one and two, but noes to question three might indicate a tendency on the part of the school to magnify learning disability into a permanent handicap. You want to avoid this also.

If you strike out twice, public and private school, you still have one more swing. You can supplement your child's present unhappy situation (or hope, by supplementing it, to overcome it) by either hiring a tutor or hiring the services of a psychoeducational clinic. Tutors, however dedicated, do not usually help learning-disabled children very much. If they go for quick results, they must reinforce the efforts of your child's negative in-school experience. This usually ends in results that are quickly even more negative. If they feel comfortable enough, with your permission, they will probe deeper; but they will usually probe with regular instruments — a "sound this out" instrument, a "blend the sounds" instrument, a "drilling of symbols with other symbols" instrument. These instruments serve regular students well in school; they serve the learning-disabled student half-well. So the learning-disabled student gains only a half year, a little more or a little less, after a year's instruction. With the individual attention of a tutor, he may gain two thirds of a year, but he is still lagging at this rate and will never catch up. Discouragement, frustration, and "quitting behavior" will increase for the child. He will sum up his situation: "I *still* can't learn in spite of all this help I'm getting. I'm a bigger dummy than I thought I was." Yet you might luck out with a tutor. There are some around who understand learning disability. But, before you hire a tutor, ask the applicant if he has had the opportunity to work with learning-disabled children. If the answer is yes, ask about previous clients. Check with these clients for results. If answers indicate that the children in question have reached "normality" or are getting ever closer to it, hire this tutor. If the tutor has no experience with learning disability, but your gut tells you to give the tutor a try, do it. Maybe you'll discover a "star" who can help your child and then help other children. But the chances are against it.

Treat psychoeducational clinics just as you treated private schools. They are expensive. Make them prove their results.

Psychologists can be helpful in identifying your child's problem, reducing family discord, if any, and building your child's confidence. But this is confidence built on sand unless the psychologist can help you locate the right school for your child — and you. Know how to check out schools, as well as clinics. And you know whether you can afford either. You also know your chances with Public Law 941, but give it a try anyhow — at least for a while. After all, in the right school environment, your child should not need much more help from a psychologist.

But you might strike out for a third time. When you get to the point that you feel you are not in the same ball game with schools, tutors, clinics, and psychologists, then you have no resource left but to become the teacher. In this case, you should study the techniques listed in Part Four of this book carefully, and, after harnessing all the determination, empathy, faith, hope, and love that you can, you should implement them with your very own child. I tried these techniques at home, around the kitchen table, with my own learning-disabled daughter, and they worked. She is having an exciting and successful go at it in the mainstream of school in spite of all of its symbols and semantics. And just as important to me, she is still chasing butterflies and going to sit on the car before bed to look at the stars.

There is a final circumstance that deserves consideration here. Sometimes a child with specific learning problems is mainstreamed too soon. He enters the academic world of "normality" only to start failing again. And his new situation becomes more damaging than his old one, for he is older and more aware and can feel hurt more deeply and hate more deeply. Premature mainstreaming can happen for a variety of reasons. Perhaps the child has reached a transition stage in school — primary to elementary, elementary to middle school, middle to junior high, or junior high to high school — at which special help facilities are scarce or not available. Maybe a teacher, administrator, or specialist has made an error in judgment, emphasizing test scores too much, and day-in/day-out success and staying power not enough. It could be that his parents have forced premature mainstreaming by insisting on academic acceleration.

This is a very uncomfortable situation for the child and his parents. The child thinks, "Here's proof that I don't fit in this wordy world that my parents and school think is so important. I got a lot of special help and I still can't make it." "Clamp" goes the shell of withdrawal or "bang" falls the curtain of dissimulation and petulance or "crash-crumble" goes the veneer of social conditioning, and the child becomes a big, inexcusable brat instead of a small, embarrassing one.

The parent asks, "Where do I go from here? I'm not just back to round one. I'm in a new fight, without padded gloves, with bare knuckles and bared teeth."

Indeed, where does the parent go from here? The circumstance should have been avoided, the mistake never made. But it has happened. Can anything be done to undo the wrong? I can suggest two possibilities. If the child's deficit is not overwhelming, the parent should help at home with every resource of energy. He/she should use the same energy to communicate weekly, sometimes daily, with all the teachers involved. Ask for specific gaps the child must fill, particular goals the child must achieve. Then help the teacher help the child. The parent may not be very popular at school, may become a splinter in the sometimes soft backside of educational practices. So what! Parenting is an intense and serious business that must be pursued in spite of unpopularity. This extra help and caring, this extra persistence, will probably bridge the gap between a particular teacher's expectations and the child's present inability to meet them.

If the child's deficit is great and persistent, if effort at home coordinated with input from school proves hopeless, the parent and child must agree on two premises.

Premise one: You, the child, are not stupid. You may not understand a word, but you understand and relate to what the word describes. There are many out there in that awesome, semantic world who can read and spell *screwdriver* but don't know which way to turn it, who can name a tree but only know it as a category or an image of past experience, not as an individual thing that happens to be here right now and would still be here, unchanged, without name and category. The words used by the parent are not important; the concept is. The child must be convinced that he is wholesomely human and worthwhile if he never learns to read another word. Then he can grow and contribute in spite of the limits that society may try to impose on the likes of him.

Premise two: You, young man or lady, are capable of learning to read and write as well as most others. If you are willingly to train yourself in this regard, I will work with you until the task is accomplished, until you earn your credits or GED diploma or simply learn to read and write better. In this way you will have more life options than otherwise. Stay with me and I will stay with you.

I suggest that the parent who reaches agreement with the child on the above premises use the techniques described in Part Four when helping the child.

19

A Plea for a New Perspective by Society

SOCIETY NEEDS CREATIVE SOLUTIONS to personal, interpersonal, intergroup, and international problems. It must find creative applications for technology — applications that address themselves to more than physical comfort, organization of data, and destruction. Just as the individual must "center" himself and find the homeostatic balance that is his natural function and condition, so society must eventually "center" itself and achieve balance. If it does not, it will someday suffer a massive breakdown. Society, like the individuals that constitute it, must generate within itself a feeling of real, nonsemantic stability and security.

Needless to say, there are no creative solutions without creative people. There are no concrete solutions without concrete people. There will be no timeless solutions until people stop measuring existence solely as a function of time.

Society has within its membership those who are inclined to perceive the world without the constraint of words and without the veneer of time. But these members are often semantically disabled; inferior in the word-wiseness that makes us most human and most Godlike.

I feel that it is about time that mankind take serious inventory of its membership. It may find that disabled members are more able than it ever guessed. Let me tell you about the creativeness of learning-disabled children.

Once, many years back, I was teaching a special class in a small, dark room. Don't be surprised, because special classes years ago were often consigned to whatever quarters were left over after regular classes were scheduled. I know of special classes that were taught on stage behind a curtain, at the end of a hallway, and in the janitor's room. We were in none of these, only a room that was too small, ill-lighted, and practically windowless. Learning-disabled children want to see outside, for outside is where it's at. They also do not like being cramped, for they are tense and touchy physically. They begged me through the month of September to find them another room. By October they realized that I could not effect a change, though they knew that I had tried. I told them that it was made clear to me that there would be no upsetting of schedule and placement. So they came to me with a proposal.

"Let's only use this room on very bad days. One day a week we can have class outdoors. So what if it's cold or it snows or drizzles. We can dress for that if you insist on it. We can learn a lot in snow and drizzle. Another day we can use for field trips. We'll take our books along if you like. Another day we can spend at the Science Museum. At ten cents a head, the cost won't come to much. We can raise the money. Another day we can spend at the library. That's free. Each Friday we can have class in the gym, all spread out (the gym wasn't used on Fridays). We can concentrate on heavy work and you can help us one at a time." I was taken with their suggestion in spite of its atypicality. It touched my whimsy, so I went straight to the administration with a modified proposal and was shot down. We survived the dark room for eight more months. Thinking back, I know that the administration was held back by cultural constraints. But the children were likewise constrained. Today, learning-disabled children have airy, light, delightful rooms. But they are still constrained by their label.

Another example. Some years ago my learning-disabled children constantly expressed a particular upset to me. "The other kids are calling us 'retard' and 'low-life,'" they complained. "Do something about it." I had enough confidence in their ability by then that I answered, "What can I do? The more I interfere, the more they'll put you down. You can handle it. You'll think of a way." Within a short time they stopped plaguing me with their complaints. I asked what they did to change things. Their answer, abbreviated, follows. It is a creative classic.

"Mr. Lyman, we just kept our eyes open. We picked out the most popular kids in the school. We hung around them and found out that they weren't the ones who put us down. They were super confident, did their own thing, didn't care what anybody else thought, and had followers by the dozens. Everybody wanted to be like them. We found that we were like them when we stopped feeling sorry for ourselves. We joined them. We didn't have to follow. We're popular now. Most kids like us. Only sick kids put us down." God bless resilient human nature and those who size up real situations instead of wordy representations of them.

Here is another example of the creative ability of learning-disabled children. Many years ago, I was having a very tough struggle trying to reach and teach Ricky. Ricky and I just did not hit it off. He would not submit to any of my techniques and tried to bolt from the room anytime I applied pressure. I thought often of sending him to the office but I didn't do this because I knew that he would come back worse than before, with a smirk that would say, "See, you knew I was a lost cause all along and you didn't even know what to do about it, so you sent me to somebody else." With Ricky I was truly up against it, and the other students knew it. He wanted help but I couldn't find a way to get him to accept it.

After school one day, I saw Robert sitting on the floor reading after everyone else had left. I told him he'd better get going or his car pool would be upset. He said, "Mr. Lyman, sit down. This will only take a minute." After I sat, Robert told me, "Mr. Lyman, you can't teach Ricky. He hates adults. But we can." "Yes, but I'm the teacher," I said. "Look," said Robert, "the teacher is anybody who can teach. You may be my teacher, but you're not Ricky's."

The next day Robert and two other boys took Ricky in hand and taught him. He responded beautifully, joined the group and started to learn. A few days later Robert told me, "He's ready," and turned him over to me.

What did Robert and his friends do? I never asked, afraid to upset the apple cart. (Ricky was smiling at me constantly and cooperating as if I were a long lost father, brother, friend, now found.) But I surmised what happened from snatches of conversation I overheard. Before I tell you, note that Robert never came to me and said, "See how great I am. See what I did for you." Learning-disabled children, in their natural state, are ordinarily not like this. Their satisfaction comes more from accomplishment than from praise. Only those children who sell out to culture and its expectations seek accolades. More than seeking, they demand them. "If I can't read," they shout, "I can still please you. Look at what else I can do."

Back to my story. Robert and friends told Ricky that I was cool, unlike other uptight adults, when it came to reading, writing, and arithmetic. They demanded that he watch what I did when somebody made a mistake. "See," they said after observation, "he doesn't make him feel stupid even if he is. He tells him that he makes sense to himself and to the teacher but that they should learn together how to make sense to the rest of the world. He doesn't make *us* feel dumb. He takes it out on everybody else." Apparently, Ricky was searching for one ally in the adult world. For the rest of the year, he cooperated with me as if I were the prophet of whatever God directed him.

Another time, I was meeting with Mark and his mother and father. They were very angry because he was, they said, "lazy, immature, irresponsible, and sloppy." "This is why we called for this conference," they added. "Maybe you can help." Then the parents took turns giving examples of Mark's transgressions and confirming each other's examples with nods. After about two minutes of this, I interrupted.

"Mark, what do you have to say about this?"

"Nothing."

"Are you sure?"

"Yes."

"NO, I won't take that. You have to say something."

"Okay, I will." He sighed and began (here follows his statement to the best of my recollection):

"Mom and Dad, you both make me too important, because you don't know yourselves well enough. Dad, you hate your job and take it out on Mom. Mom, you think life is boring. That's all you ever talk about. You can't even talk to each other anymore, except about me. You're both taking out your unhappiness on me. Be happy with what you're doing and be happy with each other, and you'll see that I'm not a monster but a nice kid. I love you, but your eyes don't see me as I am."

Some statement from a youngster who couldn't see symbols as others see them.

Here is another account of learning-disabled creativity.

A group of my learning-disabled youngsters decided to hold a car wash to help pay for a yearbook. They found a gas station owner who gave them the go-ahead to use his station for the wash. In fact, he said that just the weekend before a "college prep" group of kids had a car wash there.

The kids showed up early on a Saturday morning, ready for action. They had the usual signs, posted a few, and chose the girls to hold a few others. They waited but hardly anybody pulled in for a wash. About 11:00 A.M. I thought that they were ready to quit because I noticed a lot of whispering going on back and forth. Then they gathered up their signs, turned them over and wrote new ones. In place of CAR WASH, they wrote ƆAR WHASH. In place of BEST WASH IN TOWN, they wrote BETS WHASH IN TNOWN. After posting these signs in front of the station, they gave a sign to one of the girls and positioned her at the corner where the cars had to turn in. The sign read, HELP DYSLEƆIX KIDS. MAYBE WE CAN'T READ GOOD, BUT WE WASH GOOD. The prettiest girl stood next to her with a sweet, sorrowful look on her face. Her sign read, WE LOVE YUO. DO YUO LOVE US?

From that point on, business bustled all day. I learned later that the prep-school kids had declared that corner a dead spot. They made only $28 in eight hours. We made $168 between 11:00 and 3:00. The prep school charged $2.00 per car. We charged $1.50.

I have another example. I was teaching reading and writing "melody" to a group of learning-disabled children. I had never used the term *melody* with the group but a student sensed my purpose and said, "Mr. Lyman, you're trying to show us how to do school work with rhythm. Why don't you use music?" I was trying to build individual, personalized melodies that could be internalized in the individual body-mind and was afraid that music with its frequent changes in mood, climax, and pitch would defeat my purpose. I explained this to the student. "Hey," he said, "Punk and New Wave won't do that. It stays the same."

I had heard quite a bit of Punk and New Wave from my son's stereo and loathed it. But I had to agree with the student. It was very repetitious and monotonous, "ding, ding, Dong; ding, ding, Dong." The lyrics though. They would never do.

"Look," I said, "even if the music doesn't distract you, the words will."

"Why don't you record just the music?" he persisted. So I did. My son played the awful stuff on the piano and I recorded it. From then on we had occasional spelling and reading lessons to the accompaniment of Devo, the Cars, and the Police. It was a nice change of pace.

Man is a creature who is always trying to figure things out. Why can't he figure out the learning-disability riddle? I used to ask myself this question often. One day it occurred to me to ask my SLD children why they couldn't read or write as well as other children. I gave them time to think about their answers and discuss them among themselves. Here's a sampling of the answers I recorded.

"I think I look from my eyes instead of through them. My eyes and my brain seem separated by something."

"I can't hear something and see something and do it at the same time."

"My hand won't do what my brain wants it to do."

"I see the words but I can't picture them so I forget them."

"Learning is just too hard. I get hyperactive and angry and then I get in trouble."

"I always feel uptight. School makes it even worse."

"I can never remember anything that I just learned."

"When I try to learn I feel dizzy and out of balance. I always try to get out of it."

"See, I can't see this right. I can't write it right. But I'm good with my hands and I have good eyes. Something's wrong with my brain. I get madder every day."

"I've had enough of this book shit. This stuff's not for me."

"I'm tired of being special. I'm no O.E. [Candidate for Occupational Education]. If I want to work on cars it's because I want to. Not because somebody says I have to."

And a bright little SLD girl said:

"School mixes me up, so everything mixes me up. But I like people anyhow."

Culture and school, the principal tool of culture, should not make these children feel dizzy, out of balance, mad, or mixed up. Their disability is culture's disability, created and sustained by the lordship that society grants to semantics. Unable to become culturally viable under semantic conditions, the learning-disabled child is left with four alternatives:

1. Withdraw from society and become culturally sick, a candidate for mental health centers.
2. Undermine society and become predelinquent, delinquent, and eventually criminal.
3. Struggle for a niche in a society that has few niches for illiterates. (Thank God that many learning-disabled youngsters, growing older, have a creativity stronger than rancor. Many find niches, some low on the social ladder, some few high up.)
4. Struggle to become literate and join the mainstream of society. (This is not as easy as it used to be. Labels set limits. I had no label so I knew no limits. Today's learning-disabled kids are label limited and those without labels are limited by culture. Learn fast, achieve fast, or perhaps be lost. Horatio Alger stories don't happen much anymore.)

Culture cuts too swift and too deep. Not many can chance upon a cultural rift that will allow for symbolic/semantic slowness or inefficiency. This is not likely to change in our lifetime. But society should not, even for the best and highest motives, shut out concrete, creative, happy children who do not perceive life as a confrontation but appreciate it as a gift to be observed, played with, even knocked around a little bit. Society's learning disability lies in its inability to recognize what its "learning-disabled" minority can wreak upon it and bestow on it.

We are inclined to call the antics of the learning-disabled child "nonsense." These antics do not fit into the prearranged semantic patterns we use to overlay reality. Perhaps the non-sense judgment exists only in our minds. The child's nonsense may make a lot of sense in the concrete world that he experiences. Sense that society might benefit from using.

The present definition of *learning disability* carries two implications that can straitjacket the personal and social growth of the child. Implication one covers the child with a shadow of undefined unworthiness. Because he is bright but does not learn academically, often does not take academics seriously, he becomes a shady character in the educational/cultural drama. The fact that he is disabled by universal proclamation but does not feel, look, or act disabled (until a book is placed in front of him), makes him wonder about himself in a confused sort of way. Had he a "hard" handicap, he could come to understand his situation, perhaps, and make the best of it. In his present state all he can do is cry inside, "What's wrong with me? I should be able to fit into this situation I was born into, but I can't." One author very appropriately called him the "shadow child."

Western culture has no place for bright people who can't handle words. They must wait in cultural shadows and hope they can fake their way into the mainstream. You may say that education today places these children (all except the most severely handicapped) in the mainstream. But to many learning-disabled children, at least among those I have talked with, this attempt is a giant hoax. They feel that they are expected to be "out of place" in the mainstream and the feeling hurts them. At the same time they dread their daily pulling from the mainstream for resource help (no matter how useful the help) because this is daily proof to them and everybody else that they are really "out of place." They prefer the shadows and a hope, an eventual chance to fake it. The first implication whispers unfailingly to the learning-disabled child, "You do not belong." He has little chance to develop a positive self-image with this relentless whispering. He wonders who he is, how he fits, where he can go from here.

Implication two grows out of implication one. Like all implications, it whispers, never shouts. "You are not only unworthy but for all practical purposes you are helpless. Look, you're in the sixth grade and you're not a smidgen above third-grade level. You've only learned half of what the other kids have learned. In order to catch up to them you'll have to learn twice as much as they do for the next six years, and this is impossible, the way you kick letters and numbers around. It would require a miracle, and miracles don't happen anymore. You'll just have to learn to live with your miserable self. You'll never really belong."

Studies show that ten to twenty-five percent of our children have learning disability to some degree. Imagine. So many of our children walking around with a self-image that tells them they are out of place, helpless, hopeless. But they have no other place.

So let's do something right here, right now. The learning-disabled child is indeed helpless to redefine himself unless society allows him a new definition. This new definition must erase the two implications mentioned above.

First, it must shout clearly to the child (not whisper), "You do have value. Your kind of mind and brain can show us how to get out of our heads and into the real world. You can teach us how to make our senses make sense. Not by any lesson plan but by making your strengths a part of our whole and esteeming that part. Under your influence we will become less anxious, less fearful, less cynical, less hostile, less stuffy, less cloying, more secure. With you as part of us it will be more fun to be."

Second, the new definition must tell the learning-disabled child that he can master his semantic disability, that he can experience semantic living and all its benefits, just as the rest of us can experience concrete living.

The day, the moment, that learning-disabled children receive and believe this message is the day, the moment, that our culture will take a step toward a more mature understanding of human needs. The learning-disabled child cannot redefine himself. Culture must provide the definition and the child will embrace it.

Part Four

Rescuing the Learning-Disabled Child

20

Overcoming the Disability

IN PART FOUR, as I have suggested earlier, I shall discuss a general procedure that can be used at school and in the home to help the learning-disabled child become a competent member of our symbolic/semantic culture. Learning-disabled children are as various a bunch as the rest of children, so we are inclined to say, "Let's teach this one this way, according to his strength, and that one that way. Let's go auditory with this one and visual with that one; let's go right brain with this one and left brain with that one; let's go perceptual motor with this one and cognitive with that one; let's go whole word with this one and phonetic with that one; let's go linguistic with this one and grammatical with that one."

I see two problems in this: One, symbolic/semantic learning is auditory, visual, motor, cognitive, right brain, left brain, whole word, phonetic, linguistic, and grammatical all at the same time. No doubt any one or more of these components may be stronger than another and these strengths will vary from child to child, but, in my experience, the child's ultimate accomplishment will be a function of the weakest component. Like the proverbial chain he will be as strong as his weakest link. We can tug at and polish the strong links, but we must reinforce the weak ones.

Two, in a classroom setting, it is almost impossible to teach each child individually, all day long. At best, the child will spend more than half his time at independent study or work, unsure of himself and his results. The learning-disabled child, developing new awareness of the symbol/semantic connection, learns best, like all beginners, when he receives immediate and constant reinforcement. Frequent lulls break attention and concentration, and they render memory untrustworthy. Independent study can be a culmination of the learning process, a proof that the child can compete in the mainstream, but it is not an effective means of getting him there.

All of this reminds me of my early antics in the field of learning disability. I came into the educational arena at a time when individualized instruction was a new and powerful tonic for those of us who were energetic and naive enough to try it. Determined to become the most methodical teacher of all time, I tested and charted levels, strengths, and deficits in all skill areas for my forty-six students. In reading, I added one more category, called interest, and then selected materials and levels of materials for each student on the basis of my individual charts. I was even ahead of my time because I established behavioral objectives (I called them goals) for each student in each skill area. Of course, there was considerable overlapping of levels, interests, and goals, so I structured groups, large and small, groups within groups, overlapping groups, interchangeable groups, subgroups, and dominant groups. But, being a fervid individualist, I was determined that most instruction would be individual. It took me a month of preparation to ready my individual charts and almost two weeks to teach my class the intricacies of my master plan.

"John, at 9:00 A.M. you work in this book, page so and so. At 9:30, you take this other book and go join Group C. At 9:45 swing over to Group A, but don't forget to pick up this book from Rack B. At 10:15, go back to your desk and work by yourself from Kit D, starting at level three. At 11:00 you'll have to share this book with Billy. He'll be in Group B. Join him there. At 11:30 promptly, you and Jennifer will have to share the same card from Kit A. Work together but don't talk too much. Record your answers in the notebook that we'll keep on top of Rack A."

Each student copied individual schedules eagerly. All students were anxious to get started. They didn't really understand their individual schedules, even less the master plan, and I knew that they didn't. But things were new and crazy; they were blessed with a weird teacher; excitement was high. Under these conditions, we began.

And lasted until Christmas. To this day I cannot identify with the fanatical, masochistic part of me that made me endure two months of bedlam. Schedules lost, charts flying, children colliding, blame rampant.

"You're in the wrong place, jackass."

"You've got my book, dumbo."

Children complaining and complaining and complaining.

"You never help me."

"Shut up, I can't hear Mr. Lyman."

"I'm not learning anything."

"You didn't put bathroom in my schedule."

"Rack B fell over."

"Joe's cheating."

"Mary's got my book."

"My pencil broke."

"I don't know where any of my stuff is."

"I don't want to group with Henry; he doesn't wash."

"I cut my finger on the corner of this dumb desk. It doesn't belong to me."

Blood, sweat, and tears. Up most of the night grading papers and upgrading charts. Almost every answer wrong. Too tired to face the next day.

It is easy to say that I stacked the cards against myself, setting a goal impossible to accomplish with forty-six children. But I have tried with twelve, and with eight with an aide after learning disability became a label. Still not satisfied that the children were learning all they should learn or could learn, I developed a procedure that incorporated all the deficits, strengths, and individual needs of learning-disabled children that my experience could show me. I made a single teaching plan and used it with all my students, all at the same time. No time for inattention, loss of concentration, forgetting, complaining, and colliding. Life has been good to me and the children whenever I have used this procedure. I call it my overcoming procedure, for its orientation is toward overcoming or at least mastering the symbolic/semantic handicap and getting back to life as usual, better than usual, because the child who masters this handicap has a passport to society.

Perhaps there are other procedures as effective or more effective. If they are overcoming procedures, they should be used and used intensively for that very purpose. I will describe my procedure only because I know it best and because it has provided me with a generous amount of first-hand proof that learning disability can be overcome.

21

Assimilating, Imprinting, and Accommodating

IT IS IMPORTANT to point out from the start that I have found it most efficient and most effective to relate all learning activities directly to symbolic/semantic skills and competencies.

While, at first thought, this statement may seem little more than common sense, it is actually much more. The learning-disabled child often needs visual-, auditory-, and motor-perception training, sensory coordination training, memory training, associative training, expressive training, and more, in order to learn to read, write, spell, and compute. (Fortunately, teaching him how to understand and handle his emotions and counseling his behavior usually become unnecessary after the redefining described in Part Three.) Many systems have been devised to strengthen each of the learning functions, but the exercises and practices that relate to these systems seldom have built-in connections with symbols or semantics. It is hoped or believed that, somehow, somewhen, the mind-brain will associate inputs from these exercises with symbolic learning. This would seem to me a weak hope and shaky faith because the mind-brain of the learning-disabled child doesn't *want* to associate with symbols and semantics in the first place. Learning disability (among its many, many aliases) has been called an integrative or associative disability. I have used some of these systems and waited for transfer of training. I awaited better reading and spelling and writing. I waited and waited. Then went back to a system that I knew could ensure it.

Let me explain my use of the word *assimilating* in the chapter title. The visual symbols of "readin', 'ritin', & 'rithmetic," as well as the arbitrary meanings assigned to them, are first encountered outside of mind-brain by the young child. Most of us learn to draw them inside at will, where our central nervous systems get to work on them. The learning-disabled child, concrete being that he is, does not have the physiological or psychological (brain-mind) predisposition to do this. But he can be trained to assimilate symbolic language and become efficient enough at it so that he doesn't mind doing it.

When I thought of developing a procedure that would teach assimilation, I knew that I would have to find a way to make symbols and words concrete for my students. I interpreted their muscle overflow while reading (especially their meaningless hand involvement) as an unconscious attempt to bring concrete meaning to the string of symbols that confronted them. It occurred to me that I might put their hands and bodies to concrete use. Before they read or wrote a word, I required them to hold an object (a piece of clay, a button, a cube of wood) in their hands and perform some action with it relating to the word. Ideally, the action would be of their choice. A *tree* would shake in the wind, so they would shake the object. A *bird* would fly, so they would move the object through the air. (No throwing. More real, but the danger was real too.) People would walk into a *house* or cars go by it, so they would hold "the house" with one hand and the fingers of the other hand would represent people walking in or cars zooming by. I also required that they say the word while performing the action. Sometimes we would do this over and over.

Before reading or writing a sentence, we would make the objects, actions, and relationships in the sentence as concrete as possible. For example, take the sentence "The bird found a worm to feed its nestlings." The children placed on the desk top an object for *bird*, an object for *worm*, and a couple of objects for nestlings. They moved the "bird" about until he encountered the "worm." The "bird" flew with the "worm" over to the "nestlings," where the "worm" was deposited. The first few times through the drama, the concrete (if fantasized) sounds made by the children were delightful — the yelping of the worm, the swishing through the air, the munching by the nestlings. Then the children said the words of the sentence with equally great expression as they went through the actions. Finally, they read the sentence several times with equal expression. Sometimes we substituted drawings, including sound effects, for the manipulation of objects.

All of this was the easy part. How was I to make visual symbols — the actual letters that comprised the words — concrete? I did a lot of thinking, but the specific idea came to me one day after a softball game. I had played the entire game — hitting, throwing, catching — without planning or thinking my way through any movement. I played with a kind of "body knowing," a sensory motor thinking that worked without introspection. What could be more concrete than that? My body knowing my body without permission from my mind. I recalled my "punching out" letters as a child. I knew that I could make alphabetical movements (after all, letters are made by movement, going from one direction to another and another) as automatic for my students as softball was for me. I could teach them to "body know" words and sentences. They could learn to write as well as to read efficiently this way. So I devised a system for "moving out" letters and words, in both cursive and manuscript writing formats. It started with whole body movements, then leg movements, then arm movements, then leg and arm movements simultaneously, then movements with both hands, then dominant (writing) hand, then tracing with a couple of fingers, and finally actually writing. The movements switched from left to right, up to down, just as the strokes in letters do. Both sides of the brain would be busy.

So my procedure grew. Now the students, confronted with a sentence, performed the actions of the sentence while saying it, many times over. Next they moved out the symbols of the sentence while saying it, over and over. Then they wrote the sentence again and again while saying it. Finally, they read the sentence many times with expression and meaning. They had brought symbolic language inside! They knew what they were doing! They had assimilated semantics! Five minutes, twenty minutes, an hour later, they could still write and read the sentence. After lunch they couldn't.

I had been successful in helping learning-disabled children to assimilate semantics. They were bringing words, even sentences, "inside," but the words and sentences were not staying there, not for long at least. The students were writing both hand lettered and cursive symbols consistently the same, following the same sequence of strokes each time they wrote, so they were perceiving these symbols in the same way consistently. Perceptual confusion had disappeared. Why weren't they remembering? I had to find a way to make words feel enough at home in the central nervous systems of these children that they would take up residence there. How could I build new assimilations and associations on top of old ones? The old ones kept getting lost.

I searched out methods for imprinting symbolic language in a way that would not wash out. I searched for some time, and one day an answer occurred to me. "Eyes closed," the answer said. "Make them close their eyes."

It made sense. The students were bringing letters, sequences of letters, and words inside, but their mind-brains were not getting a good, hard look at them. If I had the students *image* single objects and words, and visualize the actions of sentences and sequences of words involved in the action; if I required them to *think* the sounds relating to the words; if I made them *feel* the directions of letters and words in their muscles and joints without seeing them, I would give their mind-brains sufficient time to get hold of them.

So I went back to work. After the students performed their little action dramas with objects (repeating often, always repeating), I required them to do it with their eyes closed. Then with eyes closed and hands still, only sounds were allowed (this way I knew that they were visualizing, not sleeping). Finally, hands were still and no sounds (except internal ones) were allowed. As before, I went on to letter and word movements, following the same procedure as earlier, except that they ended by moving out the letters and words with eyes closed. At this juncture, the students did not say the words in sequence, but thought them. I knew that they were visualizing and auditorializing. How else could they move correctly? To thwart peekers, it occurred to me to erase the stimulus word or sentence and allow the students to keep their eyes open. If they continued to have difficulty they took a quarter turn and moved out the word or sentence again. Right and left had new orientation. (Busy, busy right and left hemispheres. Work together and make this experience easier. Then another quarter turn, then another, and then back where we started. Real die-hard mind-brains that just were not inclined to receive this symbol/semantic stuff had a real surprise coming. Take your body and move out this word or sentence facing somebody else. How do you like the mirror image? The most stubborn brains began to learn with all this prodding and practice.

The students finally wrote the sentences with their eyes closed. I'm happy to say that all of this worked as I planned in most instances. (In some cases we had to go back to the beginning and start over.)

Students started remembering not only after lunch, but the

next day and the next. Now we were able to build paragraphs, even stories. After years of shifting, buzzing confusion, things began to hold still and mean something.

If you refer to my chapter on memory (chapter 12), you'll see information on phonemic lists that the students compile and remember. They not only compile these lists from their own store of language, but they chart them (learning-disabled children learn well from a visual-graphic approach), they move out the word lists in sequence, many times with eyes open (saying them) and eyes closed (thinking them). They use cursive and manuscript writing. Most of the time they end with an ability to write and recite entire charts of words with regular and irregular phonemic patterns — without the charts in front of them. Who says that learning-disabled children cannot remember words from one line to the next?

Here is an important question you may or may not have thought of. Do these children require the crutch of moving out every time they have to read, write, or spell? Of course not. Does the printer keep printing on top of what he has already printed? The children are free of this device as soon as their mind-brains can swim in the sea of semantics without water wings. The child is usually the first to tell you that he can go it alone.

The child who has assimilated and imprinted large chunks of symbolic language usually needs help in making them readily useful, in accommodating them. I use the word *accommodate* to name two functions. Function one is the rhythmic, efficient, rapid, accurate use of symbols in ever-increasing amounts. Function two is the ability to connect meaning to symbols as they are used.

The step from imprinting symbols to becoming comfortable with them was an easy one. No hard conceptualizing necessary. We had moved out symbols with open and closed eyes.

Now, let us "dance with" symbols, eyes open and closed, following the same movement patterns we used earlier.

I required the students to dance out words and sentences, first to slow music, then fast music. Hard, hard work, but fun also. The students said the words as they danced them, stretching the sounds to match the movement. Then they wrote the words, usually with improved rhythm, speed, and confidence.

I thought of other techniques to "build in" total familiarity with words and sequences of words. Students were required to write words, turning their paper ninety degrees to the right, ninety degrees to the left, and upside-down. They followed the same sequence of strokes they used when writing the word upright. They eventually wrote the words in these positions without any starting model. Hard work it was, hard perceiving, hard accommodating. It could be done only in a state of total concentration, total awareness of symbolic configuration. Symbol sounds had to be said while visual symbols were made. If a series of letters made a single sound, the sound had to be stretched to match the duration of the writing. Upon completion, meaning had to be drawn or dramatized. Without left and right brain cooperation there was "no go" on this one.

I then required students to read entire paragraphs (starting with short ones) with the paragraph turned ninety degrees to the right, ninety degrees to the left, one hundred eighty degrees, even for some with the text seen in a mirror. They had to read the paragraph many times from an upright position and from each of these other positions. Eventually, I took the paragraph away and told the student to say it; then write it. Read, say, and write. Read, say, and write. Until it was written perfectly or nearly perfectly. Punctuation was highlighted; words that gave difficulty were moved out or danced with. When the written paragraph reached acceptability, the student then dramatized it (using small objects) or drew its sequences and relationships. Finally, he read it to me with an expression that conveyed awareness of meaning.

No rest. Start again with another paragraph, a little bit longer or a little bit harder. I usually chose paragraphs from texts, starting at a primer level and gradually, very gradually, increasing in difficulty until the student was performing from an appropriate age-grade text.

In order to wean the child from the necessity of dramatizing or drawing for meaning, sooner or later I would begin conversing with him about his paragraph. We became like two people discussing a book that each of us had read. But this didn't last long. I had to test.

To test the student on meaning I would make a series of correct statements about the paragraph and tell him to stop me when I made an incorrect one. Or I would make a series of incorrect statements and tell him to stop me when I made a correct one. (Great impulsion-control training.) Then the student would test me in the same manner. Sometimes I said the statements; sometimes I wrote them. The student had to do the same when he tested me.

Next, I required the student to use semantics for self-expression. Tell me a story. Describe something. I wrote down what he said. The student then underwent all the rigors of reading and writing and analyzing his own paragraph as he had done with paragraphs from the textbooks. After considerable practice at this, I told the student, "Don't tell me the paragraph. Just write it down directly." When he did this efficiently and also reached efficiency with paragraphs from an appropriate age-grade text, he was ready for "mainstream training."

"Work more independently now," I told the student. "Concentrate on information. Read the chapter and answer the questions at the end. Listen to my lesson, take notes, and be ready for a test. Write me an essay on what you have learned."

When the student could do these things, he graduated to

the mainstream. He was now acceptable to a semantic culture. I hoped that he would succeed, but hoped even more that culture would not change him too much.

A learning-disabled person can learn symbolic language to some extent at any age, from primary to senior citizen, but the younger he is when he tries the better. The primary-age child must be guided through the stages of assimilating, imprinting, and accommodating very slowly at first. It may take weeks, months, just to distinguish up from down, clockwise from counterclockwise, before letter movement and writing can begin. But if a good foundation is laid, growth can be dramatic. These children are the true "overcomers."

Most learning-disabled children in middle school and many in high school can learn to master the disability if the teacher or parent can motivate them to undergo the rigors of assimilation, imprinting, and accommodation. They must be willing to go backward for a while and fill some gaps in their learning before they go forward. Even after they have mastered symbolic and semantic language, the disability may sneak back and haunt them occasionally, but certainly not often enough to undermine their cultural security.

Adults, also, can learn to master learning disability in areas of competence that are important to them. Total mastery — ability to read and write competently in every situation — is unlikely, but they can learn business language or technical language relating to their occupation and open up opportunities for advancement. Or they can learn to read and write specialized vocabularies that might make travel, with all its form filling, agendas, and timetables, easier and more enjoyable. Or they can learn enough visual language to feel comfortable as members of clubs or organizations. There are many situations in which adult dyslexics want to improve their reading and writing skill but they don't know where to get help or how to help themselves. Adult schools are not geared to the dyslexic. Schools that give help to the learning disabled generally cut off admissions at age eighteen or nineteen. Psychological and counseling services, which sometimes offer services to adults with reading problems, are very expensive.

Learning-disabled adults who have nothing available to them in their communities or who cannot afford what is available would certainly benefit from teaching themselves, using the procedures that I list in chapter 23.

22

Math as a
Semantic Venture

LEARNING DISABILITY can manifest itself in any or all academic or life pursuits. Learning to assimilate, imprint, and accommodate has obvious benefits in terms of reading, writing, and spelling. Its application to math is not so obvious. Yet most children who master these skills improve dramatically in math as well. Some do not.

I feel that the problem lies in the relationship between child and subject matter. Math, like reading, is symbolic and semantic; like reading, it explores relationships. But reading leaves latitude for discussion, even argument; math is alarmingly exact. For the unsure, exactness is frightful. And learning-disabled children are unsure. Some learning-disabled children who learn to fend for themselves in the semantic world of reading, where things are sometimes right, sometimes wrong (you can argue when you're wrong), cannot accept the world of math.

Perceiving numbers, remembering them — their positions and the directions and steps of their operations — can be clarified through assimilation, imprinting, and accommodation. Trusting numbers cannot. Trust of numbers will come to the learning-disabled child by making every single operation concrete from the time of earliest instruction. Every problem presented must carry subjective and concrete import.

"Tell me about your dog. Did you ever see other dogs hanging out with him? How many? Let's set this up. Here's your dog. Here are the others. How many dogs are here altogether?" And on and on from the simplest levels of math to higher levels. All levels have subjective and concrete applications. Math was invented to serve subjective needs.

What about abstract concepts like place value, carrying, common denominators? Teach these concretely. Chart them. "After nine frogs where do we go? How do we show it? After ninety-nine? How in the world can we show nine frogs and seven frogs in numbers? How can we add two frogs and two people if we don't find something they have in common? You got it, four moving things." Stay with the concrete much longer than you think you should. Build comfort with numbers, and someday math symbols will make sense to the math-disabled child who fits my definition of learning disability.

Even after the symbols begin to make sense, rigorous practice sessions are often required. After making as many concrete connections with the problem as I can, I use the following steps for quite some time when I switch a math-disabled child to the world of pure numbers:

1. Do the problem *for the child* at least five times, while I say the process orally. The child watches and listens.
2. Do the same problem *with the child* five times. The child writes on his paper as I write on mine. The child speaks the procedures with me as he writes.
3. Require the child to do the same problem *alone* five times, *speaking* the procedure as he does it.
4. Require the child to do the same problem *alone* five times, *thinking* the procedure.
5. Do a similar problem, starting with Step 2.
6. Require the child to do a similar problem, starting with Step 3.

7. Require the child to do a similar problem, starting with Step 4.
8. Give the child a sheet full of similar problems to be done at Step 4 level.
9. Go through all steps again with any problem he misses.
10. Go to a different problem, starting with Step 1.

The child who does not master math symbolism along with mastery of language symbolism has quite a struggle ahead of him. His mind must learn to trust, and it will learn to do this only after his brain-body has given it a multitude of successful, trustworthy experiences. The teacher or parent of such a child had better prepare for a struggle, also. But *do not* despair. The combination of relentless child and unrelenting adult almost always signals victory.

23

Help at Home and School

IN CHAPTER 18, I described the extreme conditions under which a parent of a learning-disabled child should consider becoming a teacher for that child. I do not recommend that the parent, even under these conditions, remove the child from school. He already suffers from his "difference." Why cause more pain by making him the only kid in the neighborhood who doesn't go to school? My recommendation is that the parent, under the aforementioned conditions, should take on the primary burden of helping the child master his learning disability during after-school hours. In this chapter, I explain some specific techniques that the parent can use during after-school sessions — techniques that should point the child in the direction of mastery and move him in that direction. Teachers who are struggling in the face of learning disability and working hard for breakthroughs that just don't happen might also study these techniques and use them.

What is needed, first and fundamentally, in our dealings with learning disability is a concrete alphabet. Only by knowing his tools can the learning-disabled child build with them. On the surface, we are dealing in contradiction when we speak of a concrete alphabet. Letters, both in appearance and sound, are meaningless creations to those oriented to the concreteness of life on planet Earth. Go a little below the surface, however; broaden our concept of concreteness, and we can make letters as concrete to the child as walking or running. We do this by causing his muscle sense to appropriate letters through movement.

The following chart is based on the direction and sequence of strokes used in duplicating the letters of the alphabet. Study the chart carefully; then I will explain how it can be used to the benefit of the learning disabled child.

Manuscript-Writing Alphabet Movements*

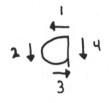

(1) left
(2) short down on the left side
(3) right
(4) short down on the right side

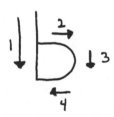

(1) long down on the left side
(2) right
(3) short down on the right side
(4) left

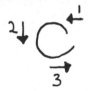

(1) left
(2) short down on the left side
(3) right

*Small letters of the alphabet are moved out in these exercises. Capital letters would simply be traced in the air with the dominant hand just as they are written. Letters that contain diagonal strokes — such as *k, v, w, x, y, z*, part horizontal, part vertical — follow horizontal direction during Manuscript-Writing Alphabet Movements.

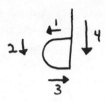

(1) left
(2) short down on the left side
(3) right
(4) long down on the right side

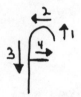

(1) right
(2) short up on the right side
(3) left
(4) short down on the left side
(5) right

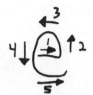

(1) short up on the right side
(2) left
(3) long down on the left side
(4) right

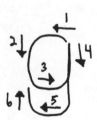

(1) left
(2) short down on the left side
(3) right
(4) long down on the right side
(5) left
(6) short up on the left side

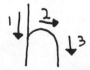

(1) long down on the left side
(2) right
(3) short down on the right side

(1) short down (use dominant or writing side for this middle stroke) (No need to indicate the presence of dots through movement.)

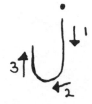

(1) long down on the right side
(2) left
(3) short up on the left side

(1) long down on the left side
(2) left
(3) right

(1) long down (use dominant or writing side for this middle stroke)

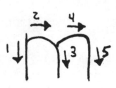

(1) short down on the left side
(2) right
(3) short down on the right side (right of [1])
(4) right
(5) short down on the right side

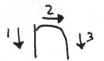

(1) short down on the left side
(2) right
(3) short down on the right side

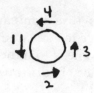

(1) short down on the left side
(2) right
(3) short up on the right side
(4) left

(1) long down on the left side
(2) right
(3) short down on the right side
(4) left

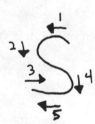

(1) left
(2) short down on the left side
(3) right
(4) long down on the right side

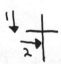

(1) short down on the left side
(2) right

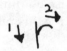

(1) left
(2) short down on the left side
(3) right
(4) short down on the right side
(5) left

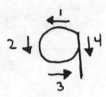

(1) long down (use dominant or writing side for this middle stroke)
(2) right

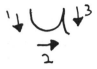

(1) short down on the left side
(2) right
(3) short down on the right side

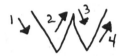

(1) right
(2) right

(1) right
(2) right
(3) right
(4) right

(1) right
(2) left

(1) short right
(2) long left, (an unusual move.
It must be made by the right
arm being raised to the right
to the ceiling then returned
to the side — a combination
of the long down on the
right side and left.)

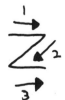

(1) right
(2) left
(3) right

Each stroke (arrow) in the chart represents an arm or hand movement to be made by the child. A long down movement on the right or left side requires a corresponding long sweep of the right or left arm in front of the body or a complete vertical sweep of the right or left hand from the wrist. A short up or down movement on the right or left stroke requires a swing of the right arm to the right side or the left arm to the left. For hand movement, in this instance, the child swings his left hand to the left from his wrist or his right hand to the right. Let us go through the letter *s* together:

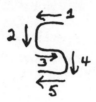

With arms:

1. Move your left arm directly out to your left and drop it to your side, out of use.
2. Move your left arm shoulder high, directly in front of you, and drop it to your side. Think or say "down" as you are dropping the arm.
3. Move your right arm directly out to your right and drop it to your side, out of use.
4. Move your right arm shoulder high, directly in front of you, and drop it to your side.
5. Repeat step one.

With hands:

1. Swing your left hand to the left from the wrist and return it in line with the wrist again. Do not move the arm.
2. Swing your left hand straight down. Think or say

"down" as you do this. Return it to the same plane as the wrist again. Do not move the arm.

3. Swing your right hand to the right from the wrist and return it in line with the wrist again. Do not move the arm.
4. Swing your right hand straight down. Think or say "down" as you do this. Return it to the same plane as the wrist again. Do not move the arm.
5. Repeat step one.

It seems contradictory that the child is asked to signal the moves of a letter with both arms but uses only one arm, going in various directions, to write the letter; but I have found that this two-armed approach to imprinting direction and sequence benefits the learning-disabled person more than single-arm movements. I am not sure why. I recall that tracing letters in big circles in the air with my right arm did not help me much in class, but "punching them out" with both hands at home, while concentrating on the direction of the strokes, did focus my attention, improve my perception of gross and subtle differences, and firm up my memory. In fact, without this combination of both hands and forced concentration on direction, a line of print often appeared to me as not much more than a series of incomprehensible curves and circles. Many learning-disabled children complain of a similar perception of printed material. Perhaps the use of both arms or hands engages more of the brain than the use of only one, and bilateral concentration on direction zeroes in on those brain centers that control perception of symbols. Maybe learning-disabled people need to zero in on these centers more directly and more often than others do before the ability to read and write develops.

The learning-disabled child will not have to arm- and hand-move letters indefinitely in order to perceive accurately. Large muscle movements help to get the letters learned, and then gradually become smaller movements, eventually just hand movements, and then finally instantaneous-thought movements that become the mind part of "mind-body" melody used in reading and writing.

Practice these movements as they relate to each letter until you are comfortable making them with both arms and hands. Now begin your work with the child. Set aside at least an hour daily for this purpose and be prepared to set it aside for a year at the least, probably longer. Follow this sequence:

I. Require the child to move out the alphabet in various sequences while he is looking at it. Change his orientation in relation to the symbols by posting letters on each of the four walls of the room and requiring him to turn to each wall before moving them out. At this stage, the child appropriates the alphabet — makes it his own reliable tool — as his muscles, tendons, and joints send consistent, incontestable messages to his brain and his brain feeds them back to his body.

II. The child does the same as he did in stage one without the alphabet displayed. Say the letters of the alphabet in varying sequences of two to five letters and require the child to move out the letters from different orientations. At this stage the child must image the alphabet (see it in his mind's eye) and also develop the auditory attention necessary to listen to and remember the letters you name. Finally, he must integrate his auditory, visual, and muscle senses to perform successfully.

III. Examine the following word categories, for you will be choosing words from them to be used in the exercises described immediately after the list.

A. Short-vowel words such as:

pat pet pit pot put

There are hundreds of short-vowel, single-syllable words. Select a variety of them for use in the exercises that follow.

B. Long-vowel, silent-*e* words such as:

safe　here　time　home　mule

Select a variety of these.

C. Words containing the most common vowel combinations:

ai — rain, pain

ee — keep, seem

ea — team, leap

ia — dial, trial

oa — boat, road

ou — soup, group

oo — root, room

ew — few, new

Select a variety of words with these combinations.

D. Some consonant blends that begin words:

consonant + *h* — church

consonant + *l* — plane

consonant + *r* — train

And some that end words:

reach　ring　held

Select a variety of these.

E. Some words with vowel combinations that create new sounds:

au — cause, pause

aw — paw, jaw

ou — ouch, loud

ow — coward, crowd

oi — soil, oil

oy — toy, joy

Select a variety of these words.

F. Some *ck* words:

rack　check　sick　lock　luck

   G. A few words with silent consonants:
      wrong   write   knee   wrist
   H. A couple of *ph* words:
      phone   elephant
    I. Some two-syllable words that use the long-vowel sound in the first syllable:
      baby   tiger   bacon   moment   tepee
      motor   zebra   music   pilot   human
     Select a variety of these words.
    J. Some two-syllable words that use the short-vowel sound in the first syllable:
      ladder   redder   riddle   rattle   better
      hitting   hotter   runner   robber   bugging
   K. Some words containing common prefixes and suffixes:
      *re*turn   ac*tion*   jump*ed*   *un*like   sudden*ly*
      plan*ned*   *mis*place   tin*ny*   *dis*cover   paint*ed*
     Select a variety of these words.
    L. Some *-le, -el, -al* words:
      handle   label   practical
      gentle   cancel   vertical
   M. Some "empty category" words:
      the   this   that   who
      which   how   when   why
      where   because   there   their
   N. All forms of the verbs *to be* and *to have:*
      am   are   is   was
      were   been   being   be
      have   has   had   having
 IV. I do not pretend that the above categories are in any way representative of the phonetic possibilities of the English language. These categories are used in most basal reading series and are only meant to provide a base for reading and writing. With each word that you select from each of the foregoing categories, require the following:
   A. Insist that the child make each word as concrete to

his way of thinking as he possibly can. This can be accomplished by drawing a picture of what the word represents, or, as I described in chapter 2, moving a small object by hand in such a way as to represent concrete familiarity with the word. The child may also act out the meaning conveyed by the word. Words that carry no meaning when standing alone should be introduced in sentences so that their meaning can be demonstrated in context.

B. After this, the child moves out the word with his arms and hands while the word is displayed for him. He says the word before and after moving. Finally, he writes the word, following the same sequence of strokes that he used in moving out the word.*

C. The above procedure is duplicated with one exception: the stimulus words are spoken rather than displayed.

*Most children who have already learned to write in school will make the transition easily from two-handed moving of letters to writing them with one hand. Many beginners will find this an easy transition, too. In mastering the skills of the previous exercises, the child has refined each letter — previously, perhaps, a jumble of curves and lines — into a sequence of directional movements. He has also learned to visualize these movements in sequence and to image them, when done, as the whole representation of a distinct letter that he can name. In a sense, he has reached the point at which his mind-body has internalized letters, appropriated them. He owns them now and can make them do his bidding, whether for purposes of writing or of reading. This is the ability that he needed the most.

For the child who has difficulty with the transition, insert an intermediate step: have him trace the letters in the air with his single writing hand, saying the directions of his hand movements as he makes them. Writing follows this exercise. If there is a question about which hand is dominant for writing, have him trace and write with each hand separately. Then encourage him to settle on the hand that performs these tasks with the greater fluidity.

If he continues to have difficulty despite the intermediate step, it is wise to stop the exercises in this chapter at this point and begin the next chapter, "More Rigorous Ways to Help at Home," which integrates the transition to writing into the procedures that it describes. Your time has not been wasted with chapter 24; what you have accomplished with the child so far will make his performance of the exercises in chapter 25 easier and more rapid.

D. Graph paper is required for this activity. The child plots his words on graph paper by selecting a starting point. Then he moves two squares down the paper for long down strokes, one square down for short down strokes, one square up for short up strokes, one square left for left strokes and one square right for right strokes. This exercise presents a number of possibilities, all of which should be used.

1. Plot a word and draw its lines while the word is displayed.

2. Plot the word (draw its lines) without the word displayed.

3. Plot the word without drawing lines. Indicate a starting point and let the child, using eyes only, determine the ending point of the word. The word can be displayed. Require the child to check for accuracy by drawing the lines after the end point has been plotted.

4. Do the same as Possibility Three but do not display the word. Check for accuracy.

5. The child plots the words that you give him, but he uses only the first stroke of each letter, or the last.

6. Words are plotted using a different stroke for each letter in the word. The child plots the first stroke of the first letter, the second stroke of the second letter, the third stroke of the third letter. If the word has more than three letters, he plots the first stroke of the fourth letter, the second stroke of the fifth letter, and the third stroke of the sixth letter. He continues this pattern until the entire word has been plotted. If a letter (like *i*) doesn't have a second stroke or (like *t*) doesn't have a third stroke, it is counted as a letter in the sequence but is not plotted on the grid. For example:

←
S i m̩m̩ e⁺r

The child plots the strokes indicated by the arrows. Note that *i* does not have a second stroke, nor *r* a third stroke. The child counts these letters in the sequence but plots no line for them on the grid.

Executing this procedure is not nearly so difficult as the written description makes it appear, even without the word displayed. The child, required to focus carefully on different elements of letters "out there" or in his mind's eye and to display these elements graphically, will take on the challenge as a game. But more important, he will learn that he can control his attention, shift its focus at will, and gain control over the omissions, additions, and substitutions of letters and sounds that so often plague his efforts when he reads or writes.

7. Multisyllable words are plotted using the first or last stroke of each syllable. Later, as the child draws the lines that check his accuracy, he says the sounds that each syllable dictates.

8. The child says the letter sounds while he plots the words. When more than one letter makes a single sound, he says only that single sound while he plots the multiple letters and always, in all the above possibilities, the child should be able to demonstrate the meaning of each word in concrete terms. (What has been accomplished at this point? Only what has always been hoped for in many years of struggle with learning disability. Total attention to a whole word and its parts and total submergence of that word into its meaning.)

V. After acquainting the child with words, it is time to introduce him to sentences and paragraphs. It is best that you choose these sentences and paragraphs from books that the child is using in school. In this way, as you work at home, you are building a bridge between home and school. Also, you will upgrade his work at school as you upgrade it at home, because as he improves with your at-home efforts he will be assigned more difficult materials in school. In using the activities described here, begin with sentences, then advance to short paragraphs and long paragraphs. Follow these steps:

A. Read the sentence or paragraph you selected into the child's ear. He must read it, too, saying each word *as* you say it — not before or after you. Do this four times, alternating right and left ear.

B. Repeat the above procedure two times, reading from the back of the child's head so that both of his ears are involved.

C. Require the child to read the selection aloud a few times on his own.

D. At this point, the child must convert the abstractions of the reading material into concrete images meaningful to him. This is best accomplished by using any one or all of the techniques that I have listed earlier.

E. The child should read the selection now with an expression that gives evidence of his understanding. If he has difficulty in doing this, impress-read (Step A) with him a few times, exaggerating expression. Then put him on his own.

F. At this point, the child is fluent with your help. Let's be sure that he is perceiving every part and every whole. Require that he read the selection, saying only the first syllable of each word. If the words have only one syllable, he should say the sound made by the first consonant-vowel or vowel-consonant combination. For example, in the sentence:

"The girl ran down the street and past the store."
He should read:
"The gi ra dow the stree an pa the sto."
The child should continue to read the sentence or paragraph in this manner until he can read it fluently.

G. Use the same procedure but require the child to read only the last syllable or last consonant-vowel or vowel-consonant combination. Faced with the sample sentence above, the child would read:
"The irl an own the eet nd ast the ore."
Faced by a sentence with multisyllable words such as:
"Last summer I had fun swimming and fishing."
The child would read:
"La sum I ha fu swim an fish."
or
"ast mer I ad un ming nd ing."

These exercises appear wearisome at first thought, but the child will probably understand their purpose better than you. He will experience in a different way the benefits of becoming master of his own attention. Whole words will become less apt to swallow their parts before his very eyes. Omissions, additions, and substitutions at the beginning, middle, and end of words will become less and less frequent. Going back and trying again will become less necessary. Fluency will become a possibility, and with fluency should come the ease and joy of reading.

H. Require the child to read the selection while hand moving the first stroke of the first letter of each syllable. In the case of one-syllable words, he moves only the first stroke of each word. For example:
"We spent a lot of time last summer riding bicycles."

The child reads:	and moves:
We	His right hand to the right.
spent	His left hand to the left.
a lot	His left hand to the left; then his right hand down as far as it can go.
of	His left hand to the left.
time	His right hand straight down.
last	His right hand straight down as far as it can go.
sum/mer	His left hand to the left; then his left hand down slightly.
ri/ding	His left hand down slightly; his left hand to the left.
bi/cy/cles	His left hand straight down as far as it can go; his left hand to the left; his left hand to the left.

I. The child reads the selection while hand moving the last stroke of the last letter of each syllable. In the case of one-syllable words he moves only the last stroke of the word.

J. The child reads the selection from different orientations — turned 90° to the right, 90° to the left, and upside-down.

Reading from these angles may seem an unnecessary exercise, even weird to someone who has never had trouble reading. Learning-disabled children do not find it strange; in fact, they enjoy the success they have when they do it. I have found it a valuable exercise for the learning-disabled child, who does not usually remember symbols, especially a bunch of them together, until he images them. His ability to rotate *symbols* and inspect them from different angles seems to improve his ability to rotate *images*, inspect them, and hold their parts together in his mind. This may seem to be an overkill of imagery, but for the learning-disabled person such overkill may well be necessary. Imagery is not a single skill but requires multiple abilities. This exercise adds one more ability to a composite of abilities that I know is needed but cannot, as yet, fully define.

K. All of the above exercises have required oral reading. Now the child reads the selection mentally a few times.

L. The child tells you the content of the selection in his own words.

M. The child writes what he just told you. Pay close attention to capitalization and punctuation here. Show the child how they are used in the selection.

Note:

If the child uses manuscript writing, make sure that he uses the same sequence of strokes that he uses while moving out words. If his writing is cursive, help him develop fluidness by tracing over words he has already written, lifting his pencil only at the end of each word. It is also beneficial to have the child write words cursively with his eyes closed. In this way he trains his eyes to confirm what his hand has written rather than training them to guide every movement the hand makes. This latter system can be slow and cumbersome. Should the child be unable to write cursively at all, the parent should turn the task of teaching cursive writing over to the school. He/she has enough to do in implementing all of the above.

All of the exercises discussed in this chapter give the learning-disabled child the extra edge that he needs to master his academic learning problem. Why? I'm not sure. The brain has command centers that activate the systematic, fluid performance of any task or any element of a task, whether the task is cognitive, perceptual, motor, or any combination of these. My search over many years has been to identify activities that trigger brain command centers ruling the perceptual and cognitive systems that deal with the symbolism and semantics of visual language — reading, writing, spelling, and numbers. Whenever I discovered a technique that seemed to make the language task easier for a student, I tried it with other students. If it met with continuous success, I recorded the particular technique as an effective brain trigger. If not, I discarded the technique as an accident. I have turned up a number of triggers. I list them here in no particular order:

— Any technique that guarantees that the imaging of symbols is taking place.
— Any technique that guarantees that the internal hearing of auditory symbols is taking place.
— Any technique that combines both of the above.
— Any technique that reduces large perceptions to smaller ones. (Arm movement, to hand movement, to handwriting.)
— Any technique that represents symbols graphically.
— Any movement exercise directly related to symbols and used for the purpose of reinforcing attention to them.
— Any rhythmic pattern that relates directly to symbols and/or semantics.
— Any technique that triggers a total response to symbols when a part is introduced.
— Any technique that triggers a partial response to symbols when a whole is introduced.
— Any technique that requires a concrete demonstration or interpretation of symbolic meaning.
— Any technique that alters the perceptual "point of view" or orientation and then rearranges it.
— Any technique that unites speech with visual, auditory, and motor perception.

— Any technique that can make the eye and ear reinforce the hand.
— Any symbolic/semantic stimulus that can, on cue, require total attentional, perceptual, and cognitive involvement.

The techniques listed in this chapter incorporate all of the above triggers. Use them with determination and confidence in your dealings with learning disability. The results you get will, at the very least, match your efforts. (This is an uncommon occurrence in this field of learning disability, where we often work long and extremely hard just to keep from going backward.) At the very most, your results will prove that learning disability can be overcome.

The techniques listed in this chapter and the next chapter suggest a method of attack that can be incorporated without great stress or expense, into any current program or approach that deals with learning disability. They also suggest a method that can form the essential core of new programs made rip-roaringly and concretely motivating by new technologies. Such programs may be just what is needed to tell a very old, very ravaging, problem that its time is up.

24

More Rigorous Ways to Help

THE PROCEDURES described in this chapter incorporate some of the techniques listed in the previous chapter, but they are discussed here in greater detail and depth. This chapter is not for the faint-hearted. Rigorous discipline is required to master the techniques in this chapter and to teach them. Parents who choose to teach their learning-disabled children may employ the methods listed in either chapter. I do not recommend one above the other. I have written two chapters about procedures only to point out the broad scope of the problem and the intensive, multifaceted training necessary to master it.

Set aside an hour a day, seven days a week. Establish a quiet atmosphere — no radio or TV allowed. Begin by having your child move out the hand-lettered alphabet. Review the "Manuscript-Writing Alphabet Movements" listed in the previous chapter. Include whole body movements if you employ the methods of this chapter. A description of these movements follows:

Manuscript-Writing Alphabet Movements

A. Whole body movement:
    1. Short down (on the right or left side) — The child

bows forward, bending the torso, not just the head. Then he straightens his body.

2. Long down (on the right or left side) — The child squats, then stands upright.
3. Short up — This is done in the same manner as a "short down."
4. Left — The child bends his torso to his left; then he straightens.
5. Right — The child bends his torso to his right; then he straightens.

B. Arm movements:

1. Long down (on the left side) — The child moves his left arm directly out in front of him and extends it to the ceiling; then he brings it back to his side.
2. Long down (on the right side) — The child does the same as above with his right arm.
3. Short down (on the left or right side) — This is the same movement as the "long down" but the child raises his arm only shoulder high.
4. Short up — This is moved out in the same manner as a "short down."
5. Left — The child extends his left arm to his left, shoulder high, so that the arm is pointing toward the wall at his left.
6. Right — The child extends his right arm to his right, shoulder high, so that the arm is pointing toward the wall at his right.

Reminder:
Letters that contain diagonal strokes — such as *x*, part horizontal, part vertical — follow horizontal direction as shown in the previous chapter.

Now you can begin. If your child is young and does not know, or hardly knows, the alphabet, begin with whole body movements.

Prepare cards with each letter written exactly as it is on the list. Say to your child, "This is an *a.*" Using your finger, show him how it is drawn: first to the left, then down on the left side, then right, then down on the right side. Demonstrate how to move out the letter. Then ask him to move it out. If he has trouble, help him. Do this with each letter of the alphabet until your child can move out all of them easily.

Then shuffle the cards, showing them to the child one at a time, requiring that he move out each letter as it appears. Make sure that you say the letter name as you show the card and that your child says each letter name before and after moving out the letter.

Shuffle again. Repeat the above procedure. Repeat again and again until your child has mastered the movements.

Now you are at the point where you show the cards, then take them away before the child moves. Let him tell you when he is ready; then remove the card. As before, the letter name should be said by the child before and after moving. Continue at this stage until your child becomes proficient — until he nods his readiness immediately after you display the card.

When this happens, you have reached the flash-card stage. Shuffle the cards, flash each one and remove it instantly. The child moves out the letter after you remove the card, saying the letter name before and after moving.

When your child masters the flash-card stage, put away the cards. It is time to simply say the letters and ask him to move them out. When he is successful with single letters, say two, then three, then four letters at a time and require the child to move out each of them. After the child has become successful at this, he is ready for arm movements.

Children nine years or older or children younger than this who already know the alphabet and how to write it begin at the arm movement level. The stages at this level are the same as at the whole body level. However, require your child to move out some letters after making quarter-turns to his left or right and also half-turns. This orienting and reorienting of direction is important. Also, when your child reaches the point that he is able to move out four named letters in sequence, revert to asking one letter at a time, but require him to write the letter after moving. Make sure — and this is *very important* — that the child follow the same sequence of strokes in writing the letter that he did in moving it out. You will find that he will easily supply the curved portions of the letters after you show him how you want them written. Then move forward again to two, three, and four letters. Require the child to move out these letters in whatever sequence you present them and to write them in the same sequence. When your child has become expert at doing this you can go on to the cursive alphabet.

Study thoroughly the following description of "Cursive Movement Exercises."

Cursive Movement Exercises

The child will move out the cursive alphabet only with arms, both hands, and dominant hand. In moving out cursive letters, the child will use his right arm for all vertical strokes, reinforcing the primary right of cursive and its fluid flow of movement in that direction. A description of these exercises follows:

— While writing *abc* , say "Left, short down, right,

short up and down, right, long up, *hold it*, left, long down, right, short up, right, *back to the left*, short down, right."

Note:
(a) *short up and down* refers to a stroke that retraces itself, such as this stroke in *a* .

(b) *hold it* refers to a stroke that goes left before going down, such as this stroke in $\mathcal{b}$.

(c) *back to the left* refers to a left stroke which retraces a right stroke, such as this stroke in $\mathcal{c}$. *Back to the right* refers to an opposite retracing pattern. Use these terms every time these conditions occur in writing the cursive alphabet.

— While writing $\mathcal{def}$, say "Left, short down, right, long up and down, right, short up, hold it, left, short down, right, short up, hold it, left, long down, right, short up, left, back to the right."

— While writing $\mathcal{ghi}$, say "Left, short down, right, short up and long down, left, short up, right, long up, hold it, left, long down, short up, right, short down, right, short up and down, right."

— While writing $\mathcal{jkl}$, say "Right, short up and long down, left, short up, right, long up, hold it, left, long down and short up, right, short down, left, back down to the right, long up, hold it, left, long down, right."

— While writing $\mathcal{mno}$, say "Short up, right, short down and up, right, short down and up, right, short down, right, short up, right, short down and up, right, short down, right, short up and down, right, short up, left, back to the right."

— While writing $\mathcal{pqr}$, say "Right, short up, long down and up, right, short down, left, back to the right, short up, right, back to the left, short down, right, short

up and long down, right, short up, left, back to the right,
short up, right, short down, right."

— While writing _ʃtu_ , say "Right, short up and down
(use this even though the vertical strokes in _s_ are separate), left, back to the right, long up and down, right,
short up and down, right, short up and down, right, another right to cross the _t_."

— While writing _vux_ , say "Right, short down, right,
right, short up, right, short down, right, short up and
down, right, short up, right, short down, right, short
down to cross the _x_."

— While writing _yz_ , say "Right, short up and
down, right, short up and long down, left, short up, right,
short right, short down, left, back to the right, short
down, left, short up, right."

Note: As all of the above letter combinations are written by
the parent, he/she names the direction of the stroke as it is
made.

The child now moves out the letters of the cursive alphabet
in groups of three following the directives listed here according to mode of movement.

A. *Mode One* (both arms)
A *long up* stroke entails moving the right arm (elbow
rigid) from the side and extending it toward the ceiling.
When moving the cursive alphabet, all up and down
strokes are made with the right arm emphasizing the
right directional flow of this kind of writing. This movement is done in front of the body. A *long down* stroke re-

traces the long up. A *short up* entails moving the right arm up in front of the body, shoulder high. A *short down* retraces this movement. In the instances where a *short down* is not preceded by a *short up* as in ↓α or ↓d, the child must raise his right arm to his shoulder and return it to his side, thinking or saying, *short down*. In the instances where a *short up* is followed by a long down, as in ↗j↓ or ↗ρ↓, the child raises his right arm to his shoulder, pauses, then extends it to the ceiling before performing the *long down* stroke. A *left* stroke is made by extending the left arm shoulder high, directly to the left of the body, a *right* stroke by extending the right arm shoulder high directly to the right of the body.

When *hold* is required, as in ∂ℓ, the child raises his right arm, holds it in position while making the left stroke, then returns it to his side.

Let us examine a sampling of four letters in this mode.

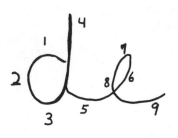

(1) Extend left arm to the left side of the body and bring it to side.
(2) Raise right arm to shoulder, in front of the body, bring it to side.
(3) Extend right arm to the right and bring it to side.
(4) Raise right arm to ceiling and bring it back to side.
(5) Extend it to the right and bring it back.

(6) Bring it to the shoulder, in front of body, and hold it there.
(7) Extend left arm to left and return it to side.
(8) Return right arm to side.
(9) Extend right arm to right.

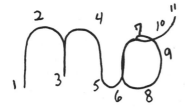

(1) Raise right arm to the shoulder and return it to the side.
(2) Extend it to right and return it to side.
(3) Raise right arm to shoulder, bring it down and back up to shoulder.
(4) Extend it to right and return it.
(5) Raise it to shoulder and bring it down.
(6) Extend it to right and return it.
(7) Raise it to shoulder and return it.
(8) Extend it to right and return it.
(9) Raise it to shoulder and return it.
(10) Extend left arm to left and return it.
(11) Extend right arm to left.

It seems complicated to follow this process by means of a written description. Actually the sequencing of movements is not complicated. It is necessary, however, that the parent or instructor practice these movements thoroughly before demonstrating them to the student. Simply place the letters in front of you and follow the indicated strokes. Through practice, you will develop a rhythm that the child can easily imitate.

B. *Mode Two* (both hands)

All strokes here are similar to Mode One. The only difference is that the child uses his hands instead of arms. He holds both hands in front of himself, palms down. A *long up* or *down* requires full extension of the right hand (from the wrist) to the ceiling (90°). *Short up* or *down* requires approximately a 45° extension. For *right*, the child swings his right hand to the right (from the wrist); for *left*, he swings the left hand to the left. The child uses *hold* in this mode also.

C. *Mode Three* (dominant or writing hand)

The student positions his writing hand in front of him, palm down. All moves are made with this hand, including the *left* move. This mode is tantamount to tracing cursive letters with the entire hand and is a logical extension of the directional skills assimilated in the first two modes. There is no *hold* in this mode; the same hand makes all strokes.

Now that you know how to move out the alphabet in cursive letters, show your child how to do it — three letters at a time in all three modes of movement. Then follow these stages:

1. Prepare cards with cursive letters in alphabetically sequential groups of three. In writing the letters, follow the same configuration as the letters show in the cursive-movement section you have studied. *This is important.* You are trying to build consistency in perceiving the letters, so be consistent. Show these cards to the child, one

card at a time, and require him to move out the letters on the card, saying their names before and after moving. He should move out the letters in all three modes described earlier. When the child becomes proficient in this, move to Stage Two.

2. You have to make new cards now — three or four sets of them. Write the cursive letters on these cards, three at a time, in random sequence. Then repeat Stage One, using these cards.

3. At this stage, show the card and wait for the child to nod readiness. Then remove the card. The child then moves out the letters in all three modes of movement. When he achieves proficiency at this stage, it is time for Stage Four.

4. This is the flash-card stage. Follow the same procedure here as you did at the manuscript-writing level.

5. At this stage, say three letters (without using cards) and require the child to move out the letters in all modes of cursive movement. He says the letter names before and after moving. When he becomes expert at this stage, go to the next.

6. Here you do the same as Stage Five, with one addition. After the child has moved out the letters, he sits and writes them. Make sure that he follows exactly the same sequence of strokes and connects the letters just as he did when he moved out the letters. Also, do not allow him to lift the pencil from the paper until he has completed the letters. He can go back and cross *t*'s and dot *i*'s after he finishes the last letter. This will take some practice, so be prepared to practice.

You have done a lot so far. But you have only just begun. You're not running a mile, you're running a marathon. Don't quit now. The results will justify your efforts and the child's efforts.

Next, take time to look over the phoneme list that follows. I use the word *phoneme* to mean language sounds that are represented by two or more letters. We don't want to get involved with single-letter sounds. Remember, "bull-enn-duh for blend. I know, there's a Belinda in my class."

LIST ONE

Short-Vowel Phonemes:*

b c d f g h j k l m n p q r s t v w x y z

ab–cab	eb–ebony	ib–bib	ob–rob	ub–stub
ac–acrobat	ec–electric	ic–vehicle	oc–october	uc–X
ad–adding	ed–editor	id–kid	od–rod	ud–stud
af–affect	ef–effect	if–lift	of–soft	uf–X
ag–agony	eg–peg	ig–igloo	og–dog	ug–bug
ah–X**	eh–X	ih–X	oh–X	uh–X
aj–X	ej–X	ij–X	oj–X	uj–X
ak–X	ek–X	ik–X	ok–X	uk–X
al–pal	el–elf	il–silly	ol–olive	ul–dull
am–camel	em–gem	im–him	om–comma	um–gum
an–panel	en–jenny	in–tint	on–on	un–run
ap–gap	ep–epidemic	ip–trip	op–mop	up–upset
aq–aqua	eq–equitable	iq–X	oq–X	uq–X
ar–arrow	er–father	ir–irritate	or–orange	ur–hurry
as–ask	es–best	is–wrist	os–chaos	us–bus
at–cat	et–net	it–hit	ot–hot	ut–shutter
av–average	ev–every	iv–rivet	ov–hovel	uv–X
aw–X	ew–X	iw–X	ow–X	uw–X
ax–axe	ex–sex	ix–six	ox–fox	ux–luxury
ay–X	ey–X	iy–X	oy–X	uy–X
az–hazard	ez–fez	iz–lizard	oz–ozzie	uz–fuzzy

*Do the short-vowel phonemes in this order: a i o e u. In this manner, the sounds that are most similar will not be taught in immediate sequence.

**X's indicate that the students I have taught could not come up with a word to fit that particular phoneme. Neither could I. This doesn't mean that they do not exist, but if they do, they're probably too far-fetched to be of much use to the child.

Long-Vowel Phonemes:

b c d f g h j k l m n p q r s t v w x y z

abe–babe	ebe–X	ibe–tribe	obe–robe	ube–tube
ace–X	ece–X	ice–X	oce–X	uce–X
ade–made	ede–secede	ide–hide	ode–rode	ude–rude
afe–safe	efe–X	ife–life	ofe–X	ufe–X
age–age	ege–X	ige–X	oge–X	uge–X
ahe–X	ehe–X	ihe–X	ohe–X	uhe–X
aje–X	eje–X	ije–X	oje–X	uje–X
ake–lake	eke–X ·	ike–like	oke–token	uke–duke
ale–male	ele–X	ile–mile	ole–sole	ule–mule
ame–fame	eme–scheme	ime–time	ome–home	ume–fume
ane–lane	ene–scene	ine–line	one–bone	une–tune
ape–grape	epe–X	ipe–pipe	ope–scope	upe–dupe
aqe–X	eqe–X	iqe–X	oqe–X	uqe–X
are–X	ere–here	ire–hire	ore–core	ure–lure
ase–case	ese–X	ise–X	ose–dose	use–use
ate–plate	ete–Pete	ite–kite	ote–note	ute–lute
ave–save	eve–even	ive–five	ove–stove	uve–X
awe–X	ewe–X	iwe–X	owe–owe	uwe–X
axe–X	exe–X	ixe–X	oxe–X	uxe–X
aye–X	eye–X	iye–X	oye–X	uye–X
aze–maze	eze–X	ize–size	oze–doze	uze–X

Short-Vowel Variants:

ac–ack–stack	el–ell–tell	iv–ive–live	uc–uck–tuck
ad–add–adding	en–een–been	iz–izz–fizz	uf–ough–rough
ak–ack–back	er–ir–stir	iz–is–is	uf–uff–stuff
ar–air–chair	er–ur–fur		uj–udge–fudge
ar–ear–bear	es–ess–mess	oc–ock–lock	uk–uck–luck
as–ass–pass		od–odd–odd	ul–ull–dull
	ic–ick–lick	oj–odge–lodge	us–uss–fuss
ec–eck–neck	if–iff–cliff	ok–ock–clock	uv–of–of
ed–ead–head	ik–ick–sick	on–on–want	uv–ove–above
ed–aid–said	il–ill–mill	or–oor–door	uv–ov–cover
eg–egg–beggar	in–ain–captain	or–oar–soar	uz–uzz–fuzz
ej–edg–ledge	in–inn–inn	or–ore–bore	
ek–eck–peck	is–iss–kiss	ox–ocks–socks	

LIST FOUR

Long-Vowel Variants:

ace–ache–headache	ete–eet–feet	ole–oal–coal
ade–aid–raid	ete–eat–heat	ole–oul–soul
aje–age–page	ese–eace–peace	ole–owl–bowl
ale–ail–mail	ese–iece–piece	one–oan–loan
ame–aim–maim	ese–eese–geese	one–own–blown
ane–ain–gain	eve–ev–even	ope–oap–soap
are–air–pair	eve–eave–leave	ore–oar–soar
ase–ais–waist	eve–eive–receive	ote–oat–boat
ate–ait–bait	exe–eeks–seeks	oxe–oax–hoax
aye–ays–pays	exe–eaks–speaks	oze–ose–hose
	eze–eas–easy	
ece–eek–seek	eze–ease–tease	uce–uke–luke
ece–eak–freak	eze–eeze–freeze	ude–ood–food
ede–eed–feed		ufe–oof–roof
ede–ead–lead	ice–ike–like	uje–uge–huge
efe–eef–beef	ide–ied–tied	ule–ool–cool
efe–eaf–leaf	ile–aisle	ule–uel–fuel
ege–eague–league	ile–isle	ume–oom–room
eje–iege–siege	ile–ial–dial	une–oon–moon
eke–eek–seek	ime–yme–rhyme	upe–oop–hoop
eke–eak–freak	ipe–ype–type	upe–oup–soup
ele–eel–feel	ire–iar–liar	ure–your–your
ele–eal–peal	ise–ice–mice	use–oose–moose
eme–eem–seem	ite–ight–light	use–euce–deuce
eme–eam–team	ixe–ikes–likes	ute–oot–root
ene–een–seen	ize–ies–ties	ute–uit–fruit
ene–ean–lean	ize–ise–rise	uve–ove–move
epe–eep–keep		uve–oove–groove
epe–eap–leap	ode–oad–road	uxe–ooks–spooks
eqe–equ–equal	oce–oak–soak	uze–use–fuse
ere–eer–deer	oce–oke–yoke	uwe–yew–few
ere–ear–fear	ofe–oaf–loaf	uwe–oo–you

LIST FIVE

Some Consonant Blends:

bh–X	gh–X	mh–X	sh–shine	xh–X
ch–church	jh–X	nh–X	th–thing	yh–X
dh–X	kh–X	ph–f–phone	vh–X	zh–X
fh–X	lh–X	rh–X	wh–which	

bl–black	ml–X	xl–X	gr–ground	sr–X
cl–cloud	nl–X	yl–X	hr–X	tr–train
dl–X	pl–plane	zl–X	kr–X	vr–X
fl–flower	rl–X		lr–X	wr–wrong
gl–glitter	sl–slow	br–brown	mr–X	xr–X
hl–X	tl–X	cr–crowd	nr–X	yr–X
jl–X	vl–X	dr–draw	pr–pray	zr–X
kl–X	wl–X	fr–from	qr–X	

LIST SIX

Unpatterned Vowel Combinations:

au–cause	oo–book	ow–coward
aw–paw	oo–pool	oi–soil
ough–dough	ou–ouch	oy–toy

LIST SEVEN

Some Two Syllable Words:

a

ba–by
ba–con
fa–vor
la–bor
la–ter
ra–ter
sa–vor

e

be–fore/Pe–ter
de–form/re–turn
fe–tal/se–cure
le–ver/te–pee

me–ter/ze–bra

i

bi–ped/pi–lot
di–ver/ri–der
fi–ber/si–phon
li–ner/ti–ger
mi–cro/vi–tal
ni–cer

o

bo–gus/no–ter
co–la/po–lice
do–nut/ro–man

go–pher/so–da
ho–ly/to–ner
mo–tor/vo–ter

u

du–ty
hu–man
lu–ger
mu–sic
pu–ny
ru–by
su–per
tu–lip

LIST EIGHT

Prefix Words:

trans–transport
per–perfect
pre–preview
dys–dyslexia
con–conduct
un–unsold
re–renew
dis–disengage

Suffix Words:

able–capable
cious–conscious
sion–extension
tion–vacation
tor–actor
ant–ignorant
ent–different
ment–pavement

age–postage
ly–suddenly
y–tinny
ery–stationery
ary–stationary
ing–singing
ed–jumped
est–fullest
er–reader

LIST NINE

Some Schwas:

hesitate   alone   amplify   ratify   adult   pentagon

You must now use these lists with the child — not necessarily all of them. How many you use will depend upon the child's age. If he is first-grade age, use only the first list. If he is second-grade age, use the first two. Third-graders should use the first four and fourth-graders the first six. But from fifth grade to 60+ years old, use all of them. The words on these lists following the phonemes are for *your* use, not the child's.

At this point, I must ask you to reread the chapter on "Attention, Memory, and the Mind-Brain." It will tell you how to use these phoneme lists. There is only one part of this procedure not described in the chapter — how to handle the variant phoneme lists with the child. When you get to the variant phonemes, say as you did before (let's use ŏj as an example), "Tell me a word that you know with the sound ŏj in it." You might hear "fodge," "modge," and some other unreal words. Say:

"Good, they have the sound we want, but they aren't real words. Keep trying."

Eventually you might get "lodge," "dodge," or "hodge-podge." Say:

"Yes, that's what I'm looking for."

Then say:

"Look at this: ŏj should be written ŏj [write it], but here is how you write lodge *[write it]."*

After this, you will follow the same procedures you followed for the regular phonemes. In the "Attention, Memory, and the Mind-Brain" chapter I mention that I also use a technique that coordinates visualizing, auditorializing (internalizing the sounds of the words), and proprioceptualizing (feeling the words in the muscles and joints). By this, I mean moving out the words. In this process, the child is seeing the word in his mind's eye, hearing it in his mind's ear, and feeling the direction and configuration of the word in his muscles. Require the child to move out the words that he thinks of, as well as saying and writing and memorizing them. He should move out one word in manuscript writing, letter by letter, the next in cursive writing, using the right swing of the arm to connect the letters, and so on through each list. When he moves out a word in manuscript writing, he writes the word in manuscript; the same principle applies to cursive.

While going through all of this, it is wise to have a dictionary with large, easy-to-read letters within hand's reach. Use it with the child whenever he cannot find a word to match a phoneme. But caution. Very big caution. Use the dictionary only after the child has tried long and hard to come up with a word himself and only after he has been unsuccessful in responding to your hints. A good part of the purpose behind this is that the child match letters with spoken sounds and words that he *already* knows or can construct from memory with the help of your hinting and prodding. The dictionary search will become more fun and more enlightening after the child has exhausted all his mental resources and you have too.

Before engaging in the phoneme stage, keep three things in mind:

1. Never underestimate the child, even if you feel that he has a very limited vocabulary. More is buried beneath the surface than you might imagine — and the constant sparring between letters and sounds required at this stage is an excellent language stimulant. Keep in mind all of the words the child has heard — your conversation, TV, movies, song lyrics, conversation of teachers and students.

Just a few weeks ago, I was starting phoneme training with a primary-age youngster who spoke very little. This child's records suggested that he had language problems and auditory processing problems. One thing was certain, however: He could process concrete sounds with exceptional skill. He used them at such unexpected moments that I would glance up and expect to see a duck in the room, or a pig outside the window, or a cow in the hallway. To get on with the story, I was going through the short vowel sounds and was surprised that the ă sound was causing difficulty. Selecting randomly from possible vowel-consonant combinations, I settled on ăn.

"Give me a word with ăn *in it," I said, looking at the child under consideration here.*

No response.

"Ăn,", I said, "a word with ăn, ăn."

Still no response.

I walked around the room saying, "Ăn, ăn, ăn, a word with ăn."

Finally I asked, "What does your Mom," but never finished, "cook in?" for the child under discussion shouted,

"Cantaloupe, an*telope,* man-han*dler,* st*an*ding *ov*an*tion,* f*an*tasy land."

Seven ăn's in one gulp.

The point I'm making is that you should be ready to expect surprises from the child as you practice sounds and words and be willing to wait for them to happen.

2. Always make sure that the child says his word before, sometimes during, and always after he moves it out and writes it. This is very important, for now he is not dealing simply with letter identification but with the real sound-letter combinations that he must deal with in literate society.

3. Stress the memory element at this level. Inability to remember letter-sound combinations over the long term is the major deficit of most learning-disabled children.

Where do you go from here? You've already done so much work and the child seems to be doing only a little better at school. A word of consolation. You do not have to complete all of the phoneme lists before you can begin to work at schoolbooks and report card improvement. If the child is primary-grade age, begin the next stage when he has completed the short *a* and short *i* phonemes. All other ages start when all of the short-vowel phonemes (not including variants) have been completed. But make sure to continue with the rest of the phoneme lists for at least half an hour every session until you complete the level required for the child's age.

For the next level of training, you must acquire a basal reading series starting at pre-primer and going up to the child's age-grade level. If possible, acquire the same series the child is using in school. The school may lend you a set or you can order the books directly from the publisher.

Start with the very beginning book (regardless of the child's age). Circle in pencil — you can erase later — any sentence at random. Then place the book in front of the child and say, "Read this." Point to the sentence you circled. If he can't decode a word that has a sound-letters element you already covered in the phoneme lists, point out the phoneme in the word, give its sound, and ask the child to say the word. He'll be able to do this most of the time. If he can't, say it for him, emphasizing the phoneme. If the child stumbles on a word not yet reached in the phoneme lists, simply point to the word and say it for him. Next follows a series of steps. They should be followed in the order listed.

1. Read the sentence with the child three times. You say the words directly into his ear and he says them *at the same time* that you say them.
2. The child reads the sentence three times by himself — a little faster each time. A pause between words can be

tolerated, but don't permit pausing in the middle of a word.

3. The child reads the sentence three times again with his ears blocked, lessening in-head noise.

4. Repeat Step 2.

5. Your child turns the book 90° to the left and reads the sentence three times.

6. Same as 5, but book is turned 90° to the right. In Steps 5 and 6, make sure the child's head is straight.

7. The child turns the book upside down and reads three more times.

8. You ask the child to repeat Step 2.

9. Now you take the book away. "Tell me the sentence," you say.

10. You ask the child to show you what the sentence is saying. He may do this in a number of ways. He can use objects, as I described earlier in this section of the book; he can act out the sentence. (It is not important that he may have to play a grasshopper, or a bear, or a gasoline pump with prices going up and down. His imagination is vivid and he will be equal to the task; or he can draw the meaning of the sentence. But in whatever way, the child must demonstrate his understanding.)

11. Ask the child to say the sentence to you again. Insist on appropriate pauses (if needed) and expression. Give him the book and tell him to read it in the same way that he just said it.

12. Remove the book again and ask the child to write the sentence — once in manuscript, once in cursive.

13. Examine his efforts. Commend them. If there are any errors, correct them. Require that he move out any misspelled or misshaped words, then write each four times, alternating between writing with eyes open and eyes closed. Highlight missed punctuation. Tell the

child to close his eyes and see it there in the sentence. After this, he must write the sentence again, perfectly.

14. Now ask the child to tell you the sentence in his own words. Don't allow exact duplication of the sentence. Make sure that something changes in it, but that the meaning holds. (Later when doing paragraphs, you'll want to phrase Step 14 as, "Sum it up in your own words.")

15. Require the child to write the sentence that he created (or, later on, the summary). Do the same with this effort as you did in Step 13. Then tell the child to read you the sentence (or summary). No more steps.

Where do you go from here? Only onward and upward. Go deeper into the book. Choose two sentences. Do Steps 1 to 15 with those sentences. Go deeper still. Two more sentences. The same. Go to the next book. Start with a very small paragraph. Go deeper into that book. Increase the size of the paragraph slightly. Continue in this gradual, progressive pattern through each book until you reach the one at the child's grade level. But remember that you must spend the first half hour of your daily hour completing the phoneme lists according to the child's age-grade level.

When you have accomplished all this, "God blast you," as Juan would have put it, "for you have done very goob." But you have further to go in spite of your "blastings." Now you must ask the child to read pages at a time (silently — only in-head noise allowed) and tell them back to you in his own words. Then he must write a summary of what he said. Believe me, if you stayed with the child during all of the earlier stages and he stayed with you, he will be equal to this requirement. Minimal help will be needed. Just be sure that you have increased the length of the paragraphs in earlier practice very gradually up to paragraphs of substantial size (at least half-page paragraphs).

Require the child to meet this final requirement at least five times. Then turn him loose. He should be able to "make the school scene" on his own now. Parents who are working with adolescent students should use all of the techniques described here. It will be wiser, however, to use the actual texts the adolescent is using in school, rather than a basal reading series. Try initially to locate sentences with uncomplicated words and short, simple paragraphs. Ground the adolescent in these before choosing more complicated ones.

Let me add a final note for adults who use this procedure. You can realize good results all by yourself, if you're inventive, but I would advise that you find somebody — wife, a good friend, your child — who is willing to put in the time to help you and who, you are sure, will understand your disability. Ask this person to coach you through all the stages listed in this chapter. When you reach the reading and writing parts, you may prefer to use materials related to your occupation or geared more to your level of interest than a reading series would be. The choice of materials is yours.

25

A Greater Sea

I HAVE WRITTEN of symbols and semantics many times in this book. I have also written of many children who find their required encounter with symbols and the meanings they create a floundering experience. I have occasionally referred to their experience as a sinking, a going-under in a sea of symbols and semantics. And I have suggested ways to rescue these children.

When we attempt to rescue our children who flounder in a sea of semantics, we should not forget that we, every one of us, swim a greater sea. A sea of existence. We, perhaps, need reminding that the human species swam in this greater sea millennia before it recently dammed off a small corner of it with the mortar of words. Prodigious events have happened in that small corner since then, the most noteworthy of which has been the growth of the self-conscious mind. We have always had consciousness (perhaps even a little self-consciousness), but words have enabled us to name ourselves and define ourselves clearly. And we found the naming and defining good. Words are strange things. They created individual, self-conscious us, but just as surely, we created words and used them as tools in building magnificent civilizations.

But the tool sometimes swings the hand that holds it;

words sometimes create the person, whether we realize it or not. Words have a strange ability to become more real than the real objects, actions, or feelings that they symbolize. And once they become real, they tend to exist without their reality base. Worse than this, they bring all their synonym cousins with them. They teach us to lead thesaurus lives. We can become so involved in thinking about happiness, delight, contentment, enjoyment, felicity, and rapture, thinking that we should be happy as well as being those other words, thinking how we can be happy as well as be those other words; thinking why we're not happy, as well as not being those other words; babbling to ourselves about happiness, creating semantic schemes for happiness that we forget the real, concrete sensation of happiness. Given a choice between real happiness and semantic happiness we sometimes choose the latter because we are more at home, more comfortable with words. People who say that they are "too happy for words" often mean they really won't be self-consciously, securely happy until they find words to define their happiness and limit it. Why do we let words control us so? Why do we think we are less human if we are less wordy?

We become so involved in thinking about fear, anxiety, misgiving, dread, worry, and doubt; thinking that we should not fear or worry; thinking how we can stop fearing or worrying; thinking why we should not fear or worry that thinking itself turns into fearing and worrying. We don't think about this or that anymore. We worry about this or that.

Words are great tools but they can become horrible demigods. They can set up government offices in our heads and proclaim themselves, echoing from hemisphere to hemisphere, lobe to lobe, until our minds can become inclined to accept their rule only and forget the reality that they represent.

We can become so taken up with *sky* as named, that the real sky loses some of its enchantment; *tree* as named, that it becomes mostly a utilitarian object for us, not a part of the living earth. We can get caught up in defining our relationships to such an extent that we block deeper, more fundamental, bonds. Close friends can spend comfortable hours together and exchange few words. Many of us spend a good deal of time trying to define and redefine ourselves, seeking an answer to "Who am I? Where am I going?" that is probably beyond the scope of words. In like manner, many who seek answers in religion spend so much energy trying to define God that they lose opportunities for spiritual experiences that come without words.

Learning-disabled children have not been blessed with the large share of semantic power that has blessed most of us. They swim freely and casually in the great sea of existence, but tend to sink in our sea. As we rescue them and acclimate them to our waters, we should *not* warn them to stay away from the greater sea. In fact, we should go there with them sometimes and let them teach us how to swim in its fresh waters. There we may learn that many of the problems we create for ourselves and others are only words grown too big for their britches.

Index